Dr. Janson's New Vitamin Revolution

Dr. Janson's New

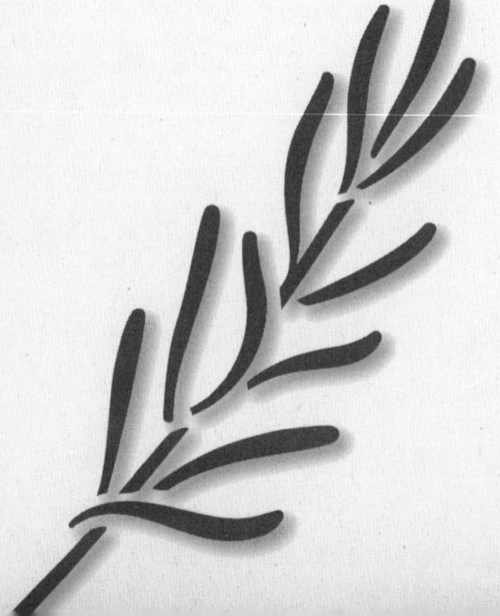

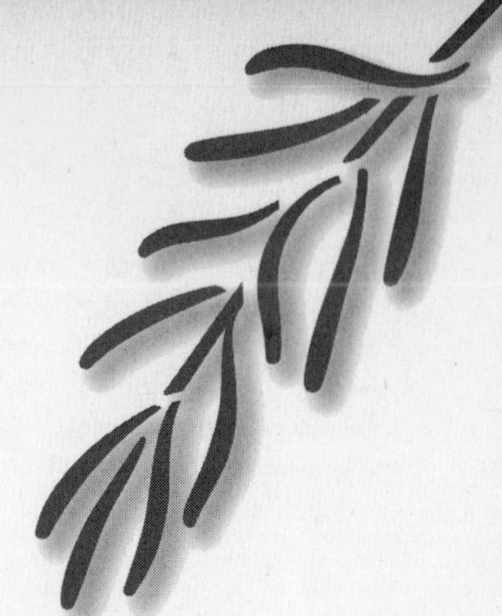

Vitamin Revolution

SEIZING THE POWER OF NUTRITIONAL THERAPY FOR A HEALTHIER AND LONGER LIFE

MICHAEL JANSON, M.D.

AVERY
a member of
Penguin Putnam Inc.
New York

Every effort has been made to ensure that the information contained in this book is complete and accurate. However, neither the publisher nor the author is engaged in rendering professional advice or services to the individual reader. The ideas, procedures, and suggestions contained in this book are not intended as a substitute for consulting with your physician. All matters regarding health require medical supervision. Neither the author nor the publisher shall be liable or responsible for any loss, injury, or damage allegedly arising from any information or suggestion in this book.

Most Avery books are available at special quantity discounts for bulk purchase for sales promotions, premiums, fund-raising, and educational needs. Special books or book excerpts also can be created to fit specific needs. For details, write Putnam Special Markets, 375 Hudson Street, New York, NY 10014.

Avery
a member of
Penguin Putnam Inc.
375 Hudson Street
New York, NY 10014
www.penguinputnam.com

Published simultaneously in Canada

This work is a revised, expanded edition of *The Vitamin Revolution in Health Care,* published in 1996 by Arcadia Press.

Library of Congress Cataloging-in-Publication Data

Janson, Michael, date.
[New vitamin revolution]
Dr. Janson's new vitamin revolution : seizing the power of nutritional therapy for a healthier and longer life / Michael Janson.
p. cm.
Includes bibliographical references.
ISBN 0-89529-993-3
1. Orthomolecular therapy. 2. Dietary supplements. 3. Health. 4. Nutrition. I. Title.
RM235.5.J36 2000 00-023744
613.2—dc21

Printed in the United States of America

10 9 8 7 6 5 4 3 2 1

Book design by Tanya Maiboroda

To Linus Pauling, Ph.D. (1901–1994)

whose warmth, humanity, intellect, humor, caring, and perseverance inspired me and several generations of professionals in the biological and physical sciences. His positive influence will be felt by many generations to come.

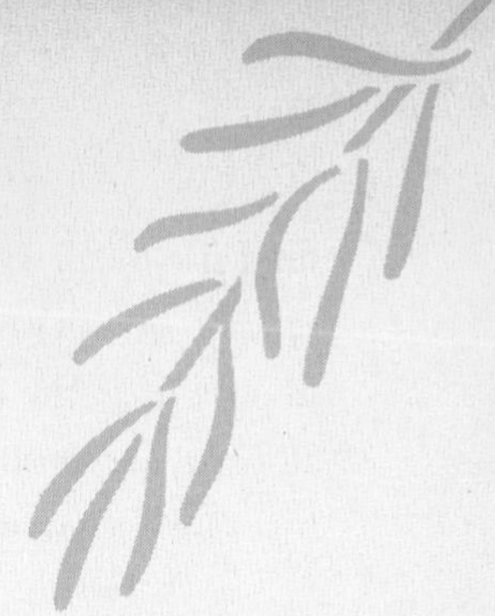

Acknowledgments

It is impossible to list all the people who have contributed to the many years of development of this book and to the updated information in this second edition. First is Kaare Bolgen, who started me on this path. Equally important are all my colleagues in the field of nutrition and preventive medicine, especially Michael Schachter, M.D., Warren Levin, M.D., and Jeffrey Bland, Ph.D., all of whom contributed to my education in various ways. Elmer Cranton, M.D., and Jim Frackelton, M.D., furthered my understanding of free radicals in health and disease.

The American College for Advancement in Medicine provided me with a professional "home" for ideas that seemed radical in the past but are now becoming increasingly accepted in the medical profession. What I learned by lecturing to ACAM doctors has helped shape this book. My many patients provided me with the clinical evidence of the value of dietary supplements in medicine.

I thank Barbara Cohen and Susan Rohrbach for their thorough reviews and constructive comments on the original manuscript. Thanks to the family of the late Linus Pauling for permission to reprint Dr. Pauling's letter. I also thank Rudy Shur of Avery Publishing Group for his encouraging opinion on the value and importance of the book. Last and perhaps most important to the completion of the book, my warmest thanks to Varuni Roberts, my constant support and encouragement, who helped me keep my focus on both writing the original and updating the text for this edition.

—Michael Janson, M.D.

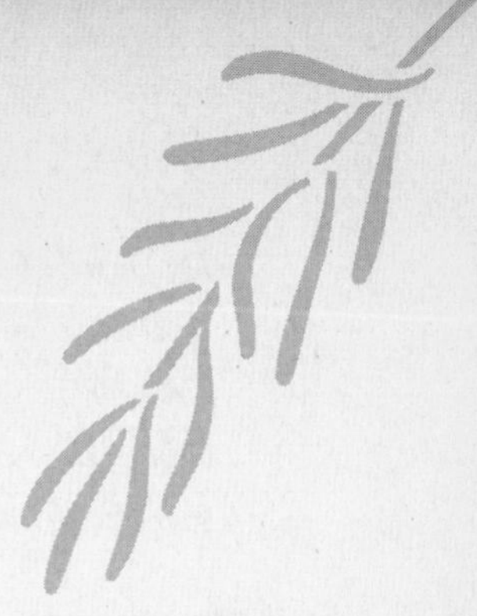

Contents

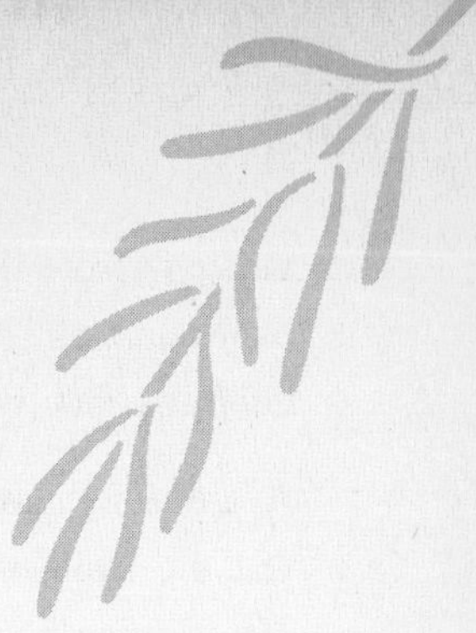

Foreword

MICHAEL JANSON IS MY FRIEND AND COLLEAGUE, and we belong to a small but growing fraternity of physicians. Of the 530,000 practicing physicians in this country, Dr. Janson and I are a part of a group of perhaps only 1 percent—several thousand doctors—who believe that nutrition and appropriate use of vitamins, minerals, and medicinal herbs should be the primary therapy for almost all the medical conditions presented to us by our patients. This does not mean that we do not use prescription drugs, only that they are not our primary therapy.

Most of the physicians in this fraternity have the following characteristics:

1. We use very similar approaches. Almost all of us routinely prescribe esoteric dietary supplements, such as coenzyme Q_{10}, L-carnitine, taurine, arginine, pygeum, and hawthorn, in addition to more common nutrients. We often use intravenous vitamins and minerals and EDTA chelation therapy for vascular disease.

2. We come from all disciplines in medicine. Dr. Janson studied pathology, I had training in orthopedic surgery, and our ranks include psychiatrists, internists, family practitioners, and surgical subspecialists of all varieties.

3. As a rule, we have very little, if any, hospital practice or affiliation. In general, the nature of our practices, emphasizing nutrition as primary therapy, often renders a hospital a hostile environment.

4. As Dr. Janson so clearly states, we not only do what we preach, but preach what we do. The reason for this is quite simple. Those of us with this inclination in our medical practices want exactly what our patients want, and that is optimum health with a vibrant lifestyle.

5. However, the single most consistent similarity of the handful of us who are using nutrition and dietary supplements as our primary therapy is that, like moths to the flame, we are attracted to what works.

The nutritional therapies that we use and that Dr. Janson writes about in this book have a strong, in fact, irrefutable basis in science and the medical literature. That they are ignored by the overwhelming majority of conventional physicians is testimony to the power of the institutionalized bias instilled by a medical education system that is virtually controlled by the large pharmaceutical companies.

In addition, for a doctor to structure a practice around the tenets of nutrition puts him or her at professional risk of censure by the state agencies that control the medical profession. As Benjamin Rush, a physician and signer of the Declaration of Independence, once said, "Unless we put medical protection into the Constitution, the time will come when medicine will organize into an undercover dictatorship." This has, without question, occurred, and the forces of the American Medical Association (AMA), the Food and Drug Administration (FDA), and the pharmaceutical industry often create awesome hurdles for physicians like us to overcome.

Challenges to medical dogma of any era always meet resistance, but never at any time in history has so much money been at stake. As Dr. Janson clearly points out in this book, nutrition and nutritional supplements can be used for the very conditions that are currently being treated with large amounts of prescription drugs, and it is a decidedly uneven playing field.

The financial power of the drug manufacturers literally dwarfs the entire nutritional supplement industry. Most large drug companies have a single pharmaceutical, whether it's Tagamet, Zantac, Prozac, or Cardizem, which by itself garners gross sales above $5 billion to $10 billion. *The entire nutritional supplement industry is only $4.6 billion.* Yet Dr. Janson convincingly argues that various nutritional supplements can be used for the treatment of the same conditions that are currently being treated with drugs, and that the nutritional approach is more successful, less expensive, and infinitely safer.

These forces are evident in Dr. Janson's writings. For years, he has argued the obvious to those mired in the old dogma, and he is doing it again in his book because he knows that we are slowly but surely gaining ground.

Dr. Janson clearly presents the need for nutritional supplementation. It is now a superstition to think that one can get all the nutrients for optimum health from diet alone. The quality of our diet is deteriorating rapidly, and the toxicity of our environment is constantly increasing. In addition, true preventive medicine is not a string of negatives, such as "Don't eat fat," "Don't smoke," and "Don't abuse alcohol." It is more a proactive lifestyle, with exercise, diet, and nutritional supplementation being used in the never-ending, yet fruitful, quest for optimum health.

Dr. Janson quickly lays to rest the common fallacy that those who take vitamins do so in order to excuse or overcome a poor diet. Exactly the opposite is usually the case: those who take supplements are also most likely to eat whole, nutritious foods. Dr. Janson also points out the silliness of the Recommended Dietary Allowances (RDAs), which are arbitrarily kept low in order to make processed food appear healthier than it actually is. In short, Dr. Janson's book is a treatise of specific recommendations on how to use nutritional supplements to nurture your system and achieve optimum health.

Dr. Janson's New Vitamin Revolution is extremely well organized and easy to read. There is obvious and expected repetition among different dietary supplement programs for specific problems because a host of degenerative diseases result from similar nutritional weaknesses. The book is valuable for both the general public and the physician. That was Dr. Janson's purpose, and he certainly accomplished it. Those who act on his sound recommendations will surely benefit—likely more than they expect.

—Julian Whitaker, M.D.
Editor, *Health and Healing*

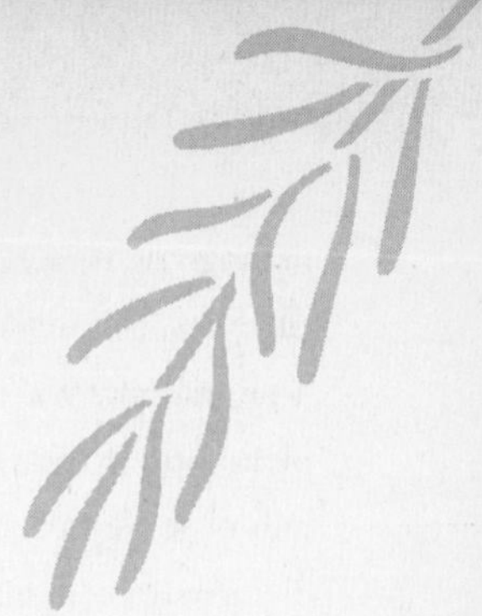

Who Needs This Book?

IF YOU ARE INTERESTED IN VIGOROUS, long-term health, and almost everybody is, this book is for you. The word *vitamin* in the title really refers to a wide variety of dietary supplements that can help you get on the road to vibrant and vital living. They include vitamins, minerals, amino acids, essential fatty acids, flavonoids, herbs, botanical products, and other related nutritional substances that I call "accessory supplements." They can help you get well and stay well, and they will almost certainly enhance your longevity.

If you want the most out of life and want to learn how dietary supplements can help, you will find valuable information here. You will find specific guidelines for setting up the dietary supplement part of your own health program.

If you are a physician interested in helping your patients with the latest dietary supplement therapy, you will find this a useful reference. I have drawn on my twenty-four years of experience with supplements to direct you to the basic guidelines for this part of treatment. (Remember that dietary supplements are only a part of comprehensive medical and health management.) As you get more involved in this field, you will find that you can prescribe fewer medications and lower doses of the ones you do use. Your patients will have fewer illnesses, and they will get well faster with supplements. If they need surgery, there will be fewer complications, and you will observe faster wound healing and shorter recovery times if they take dietary supplements. And your own health will benefit if you take these supplements yourself.

This book includes some supplement guidelines for preventive medicine, and there are examples of treatment programs for a number of specific medical conditions. Many other health problems are also manageable with programs that include dietary supplements. This is a different way of practicing medicine, but it is gratifying to get away from technological and drug-oriented medical care when simpler and safer options are available. For further information you may want to explore the resources and organizations listed in the appendix for reading or educational conferences.

If you are a researcher in the nutrition field, you may be interested to know how physicians and other health practitioners are applying the results of your research in clinical practice. You may also be surprised to find out that the general public is applying your scientific information to its everyday health problems and that some doctors are using your information for medical treatment instead of using drugs. You might also want to take supplements for your own health (in addition to the specific substances that you are researching). Research articles that support the use of dietary supplements are in the reference section.

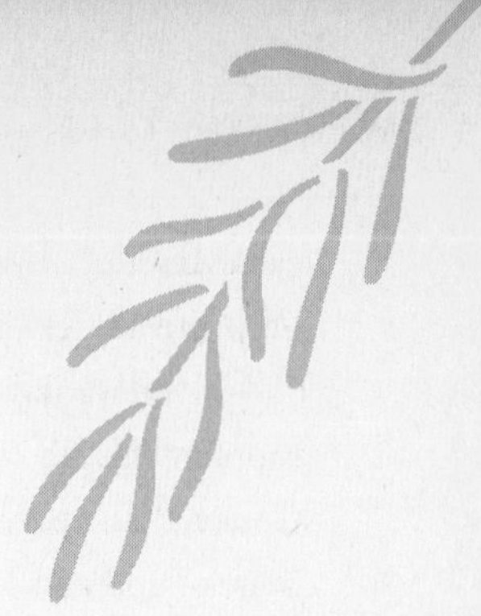

How to Use This Book

IF YOU WANT TO JUMP into a health program, you can skip to chapter 11, "Your Personal Supplement Program." You will find the basic recommendations for preventive medicine programs with different levels of protection, and some sample treatment programs. If you want to help manage your own medical conditions, you can combine some of the sample programs related to your health concerns with your doctor's recommendations. But remember that this information is not a substitute for medical management of diseases. It is important to have the proper diagnosis and appropriate medicine or surgery, if indicated.

Background information about those dietary supplements that you may want to take (or those you are already taking) is located in the appropriate chapters on the supplements. These descriptions are based on research material and clinical experience. This information might help you or a friend design supplement programs for specific health needs. If you want to look for further information on supplements or the most recent research, you can check my Web site for answers to frequently asked questions. You can even submit your own question on the "Ask Dr. J." page of the site. The Web site address is *www.drjanson.com.*

If you want to learn about the political controversy surrounding dietary supplements, look at chapter 13, "Dietary Supplements: Political Pressure Cooker." There, you will find out about the recent situation with the United States Food and Drug Administration (FDA) and their rules and regulations that have made it more difficult for you to learn about the specific health value of supplements. There is also some information on the political situation regarding supplements, and some information about similar problems that proponents of dietary supplements have faced in Canada. My 1993 testimony at the Senate Committee on Labor and Human Resources hearings on the Dietary Supplement Health and Education Act is in Appendix 3.

The information in this book is an integral part of the total health picture. Already more than half of the United States population takes dietary supplements at least some of the time, and many of them take supplements every day. More than half of all physicians now report that they take at least some dietary supplements—a dramatic change from ten years ago. We also see that the media and the government are now recognizing the value of dietary supplements, and the research into their value is increasing dramatically. The use of dietary supplements to promote health and treat disease is not a passing fad—it is a developing science, and you can put it to your own personal use to feel better and live longer.

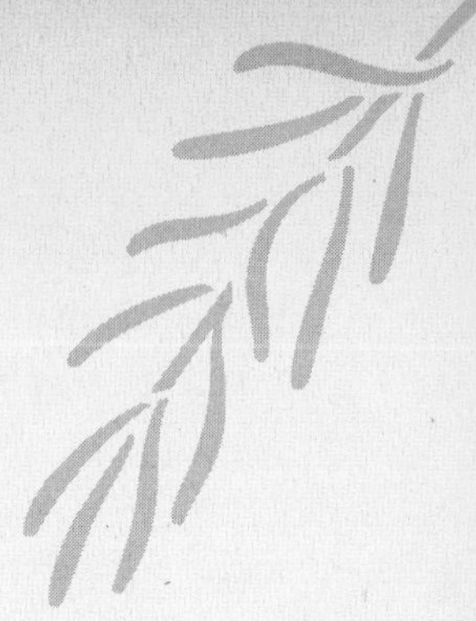

Dr. Janson's New Vitamin Revolution

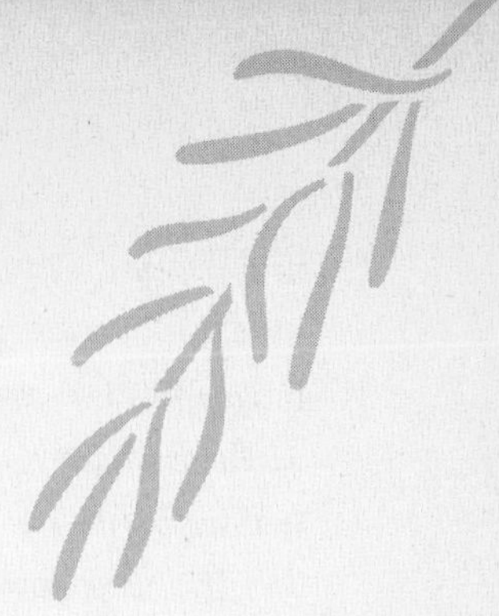

Introduction

A Revolution in Health Care: Dietary Supplements

YOUR HEALTH MAY BE AT RISK if you believe the old medical and food industry myths that assert that you do not need extra vitamins and minerals if you eat properly (what is commonly called a balanced diet). For decades, this has also been the position of the U.S. Food and Drug Administration (FDA), which appears to have had an antagonism to dietary supplements since early in its history.

In 1995, the FDA did not even allow supplement manufacturers to use in their sales literature quotes from other governmental agencies, such as the USDA (United States Department of Agriculture) or from medical research, even if the quotation accurately and favorably portrays the value of a dietary supplement. This is a political, not a scientific, position. Since the passage of the Dietary Supplement Health and Education Act of 1994, manufacturers have been able to put "structure/function" claims (see chapter 13) in their advertisements and on labels. This is very limited, but some advance over the prior situation.

If you accept this inadequate information, you will probably be left in an average state of poor health, or what most doctors call average good health. This is the condition in which the "average" person lives. You will have the "average" profile of frequent colds and other infections, headaches, fatigue, gum disease, menstrual disturbances, anxiety, poor sleep, obesity, and accelerated aging, leading to early heart disease or common cancers and premature death. *You do not have to accept this situation.*

In this chapter, we will briefly present the background of the medical use of dietary supplements and the rest of the comprehensive health program that you need in addition to supplements.

Changes in Medicine

Significant changes are taking place in health care. Doctors are increasingly becoming interested in the use of high-dose dietary supplements in the treatment and prevention of disease. They are, in fact, taking supplements themselves, even though they may not yet be recommending them for their patients. A recent survey showed that eight out of ten physicians report taking vitamin E. Researchers sometimes have a curious position. For example, one researcher reported on his studies showing the value of vitamin E, then he said, "there is not enough research to recommend it to the general public, *but I am taking it myself!*" Why should you, as part of the general public, have to wait for scientists and doctors to give you the go-ahead for what they are already doing?

Recently a colleague asked me what dose of a particular nutrient I would use in a patient with heart failure. He had tried everything else and was now willing to try a dietary supplement in the face of failure of the conventional medical treatment. I hope that in the future he will consider using supplements before the situation is dire, so it may not become so severe. Unfortunately, many mainstream practitioners still worry about the ridicule of their colleagues if they consider using dietary supplements instead of the usual medication, although this is changing.

Dietary supplements are an integral part of a comprehensive health program. I have been taking them myself since 1971 and have been recommending them as part of my medical practice since 1976. When I graduated from medical school in 1970, I knew virtually nothing about the field of nutrition. At that time, a common joke was that the average physician knew as much about nutrition as the average secretary, unless the secretary had a weight problem, in which case the secretary likely knew more than the doctor!

Unfortunately, things in medical school haven't changed much. Most medical schools do not go into detail about nutrition during the entire four years of training. However, changes are just beginning in medical education, mainly due to public demand for more nutrition information and more choice of therapies. For the most part, this is not being initiated by the medical schools, but is coming primarily from physician self-education groups such as the American College for Advancement in Medicine, the American Academy of Environmental Medicine, and the American Holistic Medical Association.

Only recently have medical schools introduced courses in "alternative medicine" or "complementary medicine." There is a demand for this information, and, once they are exposed to it, medical students often have a strong interest. Therefore, this field is likely to grow. In 1998, almost half of medical schools had some sort of education in "complementary and alternative medicine," or "integrated medicine," which I prefer to call simply "good medicine." Because hospitals and medical schools have very little experience with these health practices, some of the courses leave out many of the best-documented and most effective treatments using dietary supplements, but they are making some advances.

Opponents of Change

There are some antagonists to this development in medical education and health care. They are mired in the old way of thinking about nutrition and dietary supplements. They often make the erroneous claim that the therapeutic value of dietary supplementation is not supported by scientific literature or that supplements are dangerous. This is simply the last gasp of a cadre of skeptics who are trying to protect the status quo. They often appear to have the ulterior motive of supporting drug companies, the food industry, and a medical care system that needs to change. Sometimes their motives are not clear.

At a 1995 conference on nutrition controversies, sponsored by the

University of Vermont, three of my research colleagues and one medical colleague spoke about the value of dietary supplements in health care. Prior to the conference, the program director received a phone call from an antagonist who threatened to call every presenter cautioning him or her not to speak because he disagreed with the information that we were going to present. The director was not intimidated, but one speaker with a more traditional view did withdraw. These tactics, designed to suppress debate, should not be tolerated in America. A similar antagonist demanded the closing of an exhibit at Ellis Island that was displaying some traditional remedies from the immigrants' home countries. The threat was enough to close the exhibit.

Sometimes, antagonists to the use of dietary supplements claim that the extra nutrients only lead to "expensive urine" because extra amounts of most vitamins are excreted by the kidneys. This is irrelevant, since the important issue is not the ultimate fate of the substances, but what they do while they are on their way through the body and how many tissues they heal—including the urinary tract. In fact, a recent study showed that large doses of vitamins and minerals markedly reduced tumor recurrence in patients with bladder cancer, compared to those who received just the Recommended Dietary Allowances. This was a reputable study, published in the *Journal of Urology*. Similarly, the treatment of aggressive lung cancer is enhanced if patients are also given large doses of dietary supplements.

Luckily, I was introduced to nutrition *after* medical school and was able to pursue it with an open mind. I did not have to contend with as much opposition as I would have encountered during medical school. Since that time, I have had to learn (and unlearn) a lot. This knowledge of nutritionally oriented health care is available in the medical literature and at conferences, through numerous books, and, perhaps most important, from clinical experience and discussions with colleagues.

It is the clinical experience with patients taking dietary supplements that acts as a filter and helps me to understand what really works. Every day I am able to observe the therapeutic and preventive benefits of dietary supplements in both my medical practice and in everyday life. However, because our observations are often influenced by our bias, it is also important to have scientific support for supplements. This support exists in the medical literature for a wide variety of health problems, both for prevention and treatment.

Other Health Practices

Before you get the wrong impression, you should understand that supplements are a *part* of a comprehensive health program. A total approach includes a healthy diet. I recommend that this be mostly vegetarian, whole foods, without added sugars, white flour, white rice, artificial colors or flavors, preservatives, margarines or other hydrogenated oils, and very little of any added oil or fat (but enough of the right oils—which we will discuss in more detail later).

Total health also requires that you be physically active. Because most people lead relatively sedentary lives, an exercise program is essential. Begin an aerobic fitness program, such as brisk walking, cycling, or running, with some stretching or yoga. Try to participate in these activities for at least thirty to forty minutes, no fewer than three or four times per week. It is a good idea to work up a mild sweat but not to get out of breath (if you get out of breath, the exercise is not aerobic). Strength training is also a valuable addition to your exercise. Studies show that elderly people who do some weight training are able to maintain much of their muscle function as they get older.

Coping with stress is another essential part of total health. In addition to other problems of modern life (and, I suspect, life throughout history), most people are under some degree of stress. Stress is our level of reactivity to variations from a perfect environment, whether internal or external. *Stressors* are the environmental variables that lead us to experience stress. A stress management program of visualization, breathing or meditation, self-regulation, biofeedback, or any of a number of relaxation methods will contribute to both disease prevention and treatment. (Preventive medicine is great, but if you haven't managed to prevent everything, it is good to know that preventive medicine also works in the treatment of many medical conditions.)

Health and Life Extension

Both treatment and prevention of disease are the goals of these comprehensive health program recommendations. One of the side benefits of taking such good care of yourself is the likelihood of enhanced longevity. The desire for a long life is a sign of the love you have for the moment in which you are living and a sign of your love for yourself. Until you develop that self-love, it is very difficult to start on the road to better health or implement the programs that will take you there.

Many people who seek health counseling come with the particular goal of extending their healthy years. There are many components to comprehensive life-extension programs, and stress reduction is a significant contributor to them. Proper diet and exercise are essential to enhanced longevity, and specific dietary supplements are also powerful contributors to achieving this goal. To be positively healthy into advanced years requires that you combine as many good health practices as possible into your personal action plan.

Having said all this, the purpose of this book is to give you the information you need to start your own dietary supplement program, usually using relatively large, yet safe and effective, doses for preventing and treating both symptoms and diseases and enhancing longevity.

Diagnoses versus Optimal Health

A diagnosis is just a name given to a recognized collection of symptoms. If your particular collection of symptoms does not fit a known pattern, it cannot be diagnosed (but that does not mean that you do not have health problems). Many doctors assume that if you do not have a clear diagnosis, your symptoms are not real or that they are "all in your head." Or they may think the situation is not serious enough to require treatment. ("Come back when it gets worse, and we'll see what we can do.") This was the case with premenstrual syndrome before it was a recognized pattern, and it was the case with Chronic Fatigue Syndrome and fibromyalgia, before physicians accepted them as "legitimate" health problems. The lack of a diagnosis does not mean you are in optimal health.

If you look hard enough, most symptoms have an underlying cause rooted in altered biochemistry and physiology. Often, these causes are related to lifestyle choices that have metabolic consequences. There are many estimates that up to 85 percent of such problems are the result of these choices, and many of them are related to nutrients. Most of these symptoms can be relieved without drugs or surgery, but not all of them. Knowing the difference is an important part of comprehensive health care.

Nutrients and Other Supplements

There are approximately fifty known essential nutrients, including vitamins, minerals, essential fatty acids (oils), and amino acids. These nutrients must be acquired in relatively small amounts from the diet or from supplements in order to maintain minimal health and to prevent specific deficiency diseases such as pellagra, beriberi, and scurvy. Deficiency diseases, however, are not common health problems in America or the rest of the industrialized world. Marginal nutrition associated with marginal health is much more likely to be the problem for most people. You may, for example, have enough vitamin C to prevent scurvy, but not enough to have optimal health, a sense of vitality, and a vigorous immune defense.

There are also a number of "conditionally essential nutrients" that are found in food but are not essential because you can manufacture them in your body from other substances. The amount that you manufacture is sometimes inadequate for optimal health, and in these situations supplementation is essential for treatment or prevention of illness. These nutrients include coenzyme Q_{10}, L-carnitine, GLA (gamma-linolenic acid), some nonessential amino acids, such as L-arginine and L-glutamine, and other dietary supplements.

Besides all these nutrients, there are other substances found in the food supply (sometimes referred to as "accessory food factors") that are not considered essential, but that, nonetheless, offer important health benefits. Many of these are bioflavonoids, or simply, flavonoids. These are plant pigments that may act as antioxidants or enhance the effects of other nutrients or physiological molecules. These are often referred to as phytochemicals, which just means chemicals derived from plants. Some of them are also available as supplements, but there are many recently discovered ones that are not. (Let this serve as a reminder of how important it is to follow a healthy diet.) In addition, many herbs and botanical products offer health benefits, often because they contain therapeutic flavonoids and other phytochemicals.

Are Supplements Natural?

You may be thinking that it is not "natural" to take supplements. In some ways this is true, but our food supply is not as rich in nutrients as we have been led to believe, and dietary supplements are proven to be valuable for enhancing health, as well as treating and preventing illness. They are usually extra amounts of substances that we all need (except some of the herbs, which nevertheless have therapeutic value), and unlike drugs, they work by enhancing normal metabolic functions or protecting us from environmental stressors. We do not live in a natural environment. Also, everything natural is not necessarily healthy or beneficial to humans. For example, earthquakes, floods, and syphilis are all "natural," but they are not desirable. Supplements can help you resist unavoidable negative influences, both natural and unnatural.

The most common view of preventive medicine is that it involves things that you *shouldn't* do—smoke, drink alcohol excessively, take drugs, overeat. These negatives are an essential but incomplete approach to prevention. A more positive view is that of being an active participant in your own health promotion program. Supplementing your diet is one way to actively promote your own wellness, create vitality, and enhance longevity. Dietary supplements have worked for many people for many years. Take my word for it, they can work for you too.

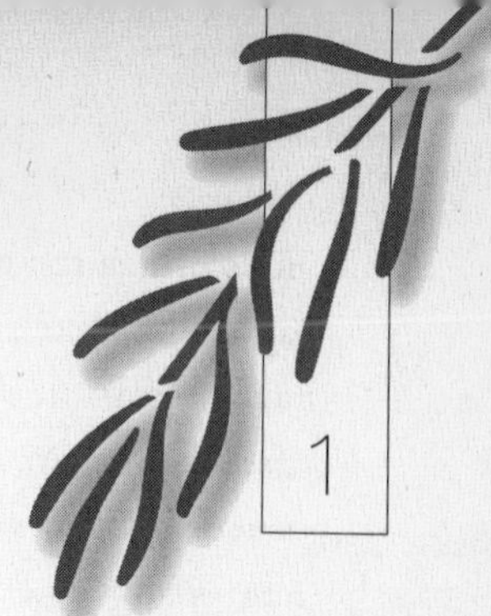

1

Why You Need Vitamins

ALONG WITH THE MANY PEOPLE I encounter in my medical practice and my lectures, you too may wonder, "Why do I need to take supplements?" Many people think—and some conservative nutritionists would agree with them—that following a balanced diet provides all the vitamins they need. This is simply not so. Everyone's idea of a balanced diet, even among experts, is different, and it may vary greatly from the scientifically based recommendations of a contemporary nutritionist or nutritionally oriented physician. In order to answer the question, we need to explore a number of different but equally important personal and ecological considerations: genetics, environment, agriculture, stress, health history, and of course, your desire for a vigorous and lively health future.

The Important Role of Genetics

Throughout all species there is wide variation in genetic makeup. This variation includes differing abilities to survive in a given nutritional environment. In other words, in order to thrive, one animal may require much more of a particular nutrient than another animal. Dr. Roger Williams, author of *Biochemical Individuality* and discoverer of many vitamins, including pantothenic acid, has shown in experiments with rats that after five generations of inbreeding, littermates, which are very close genetically, can vary in nutrient needs up to forty times for particular nutrients. In other words, one may need 2.5 milligrams (mg) of pantothenic acid (vitamin B_5) and another may need 100 mg for the same level of vitality, physical endurance, and life span. There is an even greater variation in human beings, as we have a greater genetic diversity than other species.

In the natural course of events, species develop (or evolve) when those animals with greater nutritional needs fail to survive or to reproduce as well as those with lesser needs. Except in a few known genetic disorders, we cannot determine subtle variations in nutritional needs for human beings. It is therefore wise to make sure that our internal environment (including all cells, tissues and organs) is abundantly supplied with all the nutrients. "Biochemical individuality" is Dr. Williams's term for the basic principle of varied individual needs.

In tissue cultures (cells growing in laboratories) the culture medium is made quite rich in all the required nutrients. If the cells were only given minimum requirements, some cells would not thrive and researchers would risk losing the cell line. In human beings the blood plasma provides nourishment for the cells, and needs a constant and abundant supply of all the nutrients. This requires both a healthy diet and supplements.

Supplements enhance a healthy diet; they are not a substitute for it. Some antagonists to the use of dietary supplements have said that people will get a false sense of security if they use supplements, and as a result they will not seek out the healthiest foods. It is my experience, on the contrary, that the people who elect to use supplements are usually the ones who also follow a healthier diet. These antagonists are usually the same people who defend the highly processed, Westernized, or "industrial" diet that is a prime cause of degenerative disease and chronic health problems.

Our Risky Environment

Another reason you will benefit from dietary supplements is the poor quality of the environment in which we live. Whether it is toxins in food, water, and air or other exposures such as mercury in dental fillings or aluminum in cookware and antiperspirants, our bodies have an excessive burden to overcome. This environmental burden taxes our detoxification capacity and may lead to many health problems.

You already know that the air is polluted. Everybody is subjected to toxic exposure from a wide variety of pollutants in the air they breathe. Among the many toxins in the air are:

1. Carbon monoxide and lead from fuel exhaust (most of the lead has been reduced in the United States, but it is still found elsewhere)
2. Hydrocarbon pollutants from industrial waste
3. By-products from the burning of fossil fuels
4. Radiation leakage from nuclear power plants and possibly radon in the home. Radiation, like radon gas, is a contaminant that cannot be seen, smelled, or tasted and is therefore more insidious than some of the more familiar pollutants.
5. Lead, cadmium, and other toxic heavy metals that are enzyme and nerve poisons

Unfortunately, most municipal tap water contains more than water. It is often contaminated with toxic heavy metals such as lead or cadmium or with added fluoride (associated with an increased risk of cancer, digestive disorders, and kidney disease). Often, industrial chemicals and wastes, cleaning solvents, pesticides and other farm chemicals have seeped through the soil to contaminate the water table. Volatile chemicals (those hydrocarbons that readily vaporize) can combine with chlorine to form even more toxic products.

You may be familiar with the toxic chemical water contamination in Woburn, Massachusetts, which led to increases in childhood leukemia.

(The book by Jonathan Harr, *A Civil Action,* and the film of the same name detail those events.) Other examples abound. I recommend that you use spring water or filtered water—solid carbon-block filters or reverse osmosis filters are the best—for all drinking and cooking needs. Unfortunately, in spite of home filtration or spring water for personal use, there is always some exposure to tap water, such as when you eat at restaurants or buy prepared foods, or when you shower and breathe the vaporized volatile chemicals. (At one water-testing lab, the joke about their municipal water was that it was "safe" to drink, but for goodness' sake don't smoke in the shower!)

Cigarette smoke exposure in smokers and nonsmokers (sidestream smoke—the uninhaled pollutants from the end of the cigarette—and secondhand smoke are also highly toxic) creates further health risks. This and most pollutants lead to an increase of high-energy molecular fragments known as *free radicals.* These free radicals can severely damage tissues, destroy nutrients, and lead to premature aging, heart disease, and cancer. All these environmental problems increase your need for nutrients, and many supplements can help control the damage of toxic exposures.

The Damage from Free Radicals

In the normal course of metabolism, your body produces small, high-energy particles that have a single electron in their outer shell (such molecules are unstable because electrons prefer to be paired). These are called free radicals, and they can be very damaging in their search for another electron. Free radicals derived from oxygen are the most abundant and damaging of the species. Not all free radicals are harmful, as many take part in essential physiological reactions.

Many of these free radicals are normally channeled into energy production. In some cells they may be used as the weapons to kill viruses and bacteria. Unfortunately, if too many of them or the wrong ones are produced, their extremely high energy can also be damaging to normal tissues. Free radicals disrupt the normal production of DNA (the genetic material) and alter the lipids (fats) in cell membranes. They also affect the blood vessels and the production of prostaglandins. (Prostaglandins are hormonelike substances that regulate many physiological functions, and their production is very sensitive to many metabolic influences.) Free radicals damage the lining cell layer in the arteries and disrupt the normal activity of the vessel wall.

We are also exposed to free radicals that are found in the environment or generated by exposure to environmental chemicals. There are many sources of excess free-radical exposure. They include: cigarette smoke; air pollution; some highly processed foods and food additives; ultraviolet sunlight and radiation; processed oils such as commercial vegetable oils, margarines, and shortenings; charcoal-broiled foods and any charred or burned foods; certain metals (excess iron is an example); pesticides; and some prescription medications. Many of the chemicals found in municipal water supplies are toxic because they generate free radicals. It is good to drink a lot of water but to avoid tap water as much as possible. Remember to use spring water or filtered water as mentioned above.

Recently, it has been confirmed that excessive accumulation of iron, common in meat-eating populations, may be a highly significant risk factor in the development of heart disease, although not as high a risk factor as smoking. This is probably due to this *transition metal* (a metal that can exist in multiple electronic states) being a generator of free radicals. Therefore, it is also a probable risk factor for cancer. Unless you have a demonstrated need for iron, it is a good idea to avoid supplements that contain it, although these studies were *not* done with iron supplements, and some researchers suggest it is only the meat, not the iron, that is responsible for increased risks.

By making careful lifestyle choices, you can avoid some of these free-radical sources and you can counter the others. By making these choices for yourself you can slow down the aging process, decrease the risk of cancer and heart disease, and promote high energy and a vital, healthy feeling of well-being. One way you can protect yourself from free-radical damage is to take dietary supplements. The chapters on the individual supplements contain more specific information.

We need extra supplies of those nutrients destroyed by toxins and those that help to prevent the harmful effects of these foreign chemicals. Specifically, vitamins A, C, E, and carotenoids; the trace minerals selenium and zinc; and accessory food factors, such as bioflavonoids and coenzyme

Q_{10}, all help to scavenge free radicals through antioxidant activity. They help prevent cancer, heart disease, premature aging, and tissue degeneration. Many herbs also help in the fight against excess free radicals.

Destructive Agricultural Practices

Modern agricultural practices have adversely affected the quality of our food supply. Growing foods with methods designed to increase quantity or to facilitate transportation and storage (such as the development of sturdy, square tomatoes) is often detrimental to their nutritional value. Nutritional value is rarely considered when developers play with the genetics of plants or soil modifications.

Soil quality has been degraded through modern farming methods. Most chemical fertilizers do not replace all the minerals needed for human nutrition. Organic foods are of better quality and safer than conventionally grown foods. They are free of the pesticides, herbicides, and thousands of other risky chemicals that are added to foods during processing. There is also wide variation in the natural mineral content of the soil. For example, in northeastern states (and elsewhere) the soil has a very low selenium content. Selenium is important for protection from heart disease and cancer. In spite of a diet that includes foods from many geographic areas, research has shown that people living in regions with low soil selenium have a higher risk of cancer. Although selenium, as well as chromium and iodine are essential for human nutrition, they are not required for growing healthy plants. They are rarely added to the soil for agricultural purposes.

Foods are often picked before they are ripe and allowed to ripen in transit, at the market, or during home storage. They do not acquire their full complement of minerals and vitamins, which frequently increase greatly during the later stages of growth.

In addition, transportation and storage of foods, whether in the market or at home, allows time for nutrients to deteriorate. Fruits and vegetables can lose significant amounts of vitamin C after three days in cold storage, and even more at room temperature. Dried fruits can also lose vitamins A, C, and E if exposed to oxygen and light. This is not to say that stored foods are of no value, but the lower nutrient content increases the importance of taking supplements. Irradiation of foods for preservation creates further problems, such as "unique radiolytic products" that may be detrimental to your health.

You can overcome some of these problems if you grow your own food or buy organically grown fruits and vegetables (which are generally fresher because they cannot be stored as long). Commercial fruits and vegetables are frequently sprayed with chemicals. Many of these substances are harmful, and they accumulate in body fat, with deleterious health effects over the years. A good example is DDT, which is still present in human fat tissue although its use was finally banned years ago in the United States long after its toxicity to humans and the environment was clearly evident. The toxicity problems from DDT were written up in Rachel Carson's *Silent Spring.*

Many of the pesticides prohibited in the United States have been freely sold to developing countries, which then export foods to the U.S.—in what some critics have called "the circle of poison." Controls on the use of pesticides and other chemicals are not strict in many of these countries. The workers who apply these chemicals frequently have diseases that are the result of their high exposures. Certain nutritional supplements can help counter the ill effects of many of these poisons. They include vitamins C, E, and B complex, carotenoids, bioflavonoids, and others. Of course, it is also wise to choose untreated foods as much as possible.

The recent introduction of genetically modified foods has added another dimension to the potential risks from nonorganic foods. No one yet knows whether these foods are safe, and many scientists (other than those who work for the food processors and agribusiness) have argued that we do not know enough to allow these products into the food supply. At the very least, most grass-roots organizers and the health food industry want to prevent these products from being called organic, and to have the products appropriately labeled. Some of the genetic modifications are designed to make the plants more resistant to pesticides, so that they will be unharmed by excessive spraying. Some have been modified to give them the genes for natural pest resistance, which might lead to the pests becoming resistant to the natural controls.

Stress Increases Needs

Although we seem to live in a time of great stress, I believe that this is not unique to our age. There have always been many stressors that have adversely influenced human health. Earlier generations did not have the advantage of high-dose nutrients to help diminish the toll of these stressors in their lives.

Stress, whether emotional or physical or due to injury or illness, depletes the body of nutrients, especially vitamin C, the B-complex vitamins, and zinc. Vitamin B_6 and pantothenic acid are also particularly important in times of stress. Ginseng appears to help as a tonic when the body is depleted by stressful situations. Supplements of vitamins C and E and the trace mineral zinc promote the healing process. A comprehensive approach to good health includes practices that aid in stress management, regular exercise, and proper diet. Diet and nutritional supplements provide the building blocks to form a healthier, more vital organism.

Health History

You may have heard of someone's grandparent who lived to a ripe old age with little attention to diet or nutritional supplements. This is quite possible. However, it is important to realize that potential human life span is well over 100 years. Living to 80 or 90 years may result from growing up with cleaner air and water, fresher food, fewer chemical exposures, and lesser availability of highly processed foods. Also, many people who survive a long time have numerous health problems. In spite of these occasional reports of elderly people who have not followed good health habits, we are seeing more frequent and earlier degenerative diseases. Remember, the quality of life is more important than the quantity. Dietary supplements can promote what most of us would prefer—good health and vigor in all stages of life, including later years.

There is great individual genetic variation. You may have inherited a strong constitution, but is it really wise to wait forty or fifty years to find out? Nutritional supplements help people who have greater genetically determined needs to remain vigorous and active well into old age. Many poor health habits, such as consumption of sweets, alcohol, caffeine, highly processed foods and artificial food additives, lack of exercise, and high stress all increase nutrient needs. The typical American diet is a sad joke. It would be hard to design a diet that could do more harm to health than the one most Americans follow every day.

Stress reduction, relaxation techniques, body therapies, and exercise programs are part of good health, but nutritional supplementation is also extremely important to the comprehensive approach to health care and preventive medicine. Specific chronic and acute illnesses can be treated with large doses of nutrient supplements. They can usually reduce or eliminate the need for drugs or surgery.

Your Health Future

After considering all these issues, the last and perhaps most important point is that your future health depends on a number of your current health practices—which you have the power to change. Taking dietary supplements of any kind will almost certainly help you overcome many of your current health problems and enhance your energy. And they will protect you from disease and degeneration well into a vital, vigorous, and healthy future.

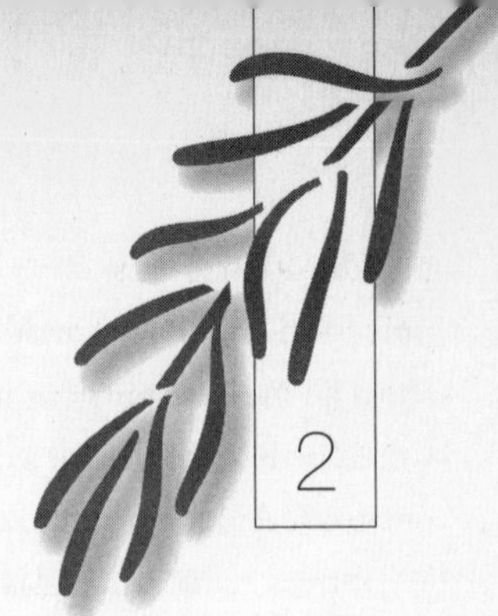

2

"Orthomolecular" Medicine: The Right Molecules in the Right Amounts

ORTHOMOLECULAR MEDICINE is the restoration and maintenance of health through the administration of adequate amounts of substances that are normally present in the body. "Ortho" means correct, and "molecular" refers to the various combinations of atoms that are the basic building blocks of chemical substances, including nutrients. Thus, orthomolecular medicine simply refers to creating the correct chemical balance in the body through the administration of those physiological substances normally present in the body, such as vitamins, minerals, amino acids, essential fatty acids, accessory food factors, hormones, and related molecules. Two-time Nobel Prize winner Linus Pauling, one of the leading molecular chemists of the century, established this definition of orthomolecular medicine in 1968 to describe more accurately what had been called "megavitamin therapy." Pauling devoted his later years to research into molecular chemistry, and he founded the Linus Pauling Institute to continue this research.

Drs. Abram Hoffer and Humphrey Osmond first used orthomolecular treatment in the early 1950s for the treatment of mental illness. The success rate varied, but high doses of niacin (vitamin B_3) helped a significant number of their patients with schizophrenia. Vitamin C, pyridoxine (vitamin B_6), magnesium, and zinc were later added to typical orthomolecular programs for the treatment of mental illness. Interestingly, Hoffer and Osmond did the first double-blind studies in psychiatry. Double-blind studies have since become one standard for medical research (although other research methods also provide valuable information. Current psychiatric treatment with the powerful phenothiazine drugs was in its infancy at that time.

The substances used in orthomolecular medicine may be nutrients or molecules manufactured in the body, such as hormones, or accessory food factors, such as bioflavonoids, that are in many foods and herbs. Orthomolecular physicians are more cautious in their use of hormone supplements, such as DHEA, thyroid, cortisone, estrogens, or melatonin, because of their potent effects and sometimes greater risk of side effects compared with vitamins and minerals. (DHEA and melatonin have been shown to be quite safe even in very large doses. Although natural hormones are usually much safer than the synthetics that are commonly used in medicine, with melatonin the synthetic is safer.) They will frequently use some herbs or botanical remedies and other natural products for treatment whenever they provide margins of safety and effectiveness that are significantly better than medications—which is usual.

Do No Harm

The first principle of medical ethics is "Do no harm." Unfortunately, the bulk of medical practice today is based on drug therapy and surgery, which are frequently harmful, although sometimes necessary. The sad fact is that more people die in any one year from the side effects of prescribed medication than from car accidents, and this is when the drugs are taken as directed. Prescription medication is between the fourth and sixth leading cause of death in the United States. For most nutritional supplements, the doses used for treatment and prevention are far lower than the doses that may be harmful. In fact, only a few of them have any potential toxicity. Vitamin C, for example, can be and has been taken in enormous doses (over

80–100 g) without significant side effects. (You might get some diarrhea if you take large amounts, but lowering the dose easily controls this, and it is not serious.) No matter how much vitamin C you take, it is probably safer than the water with which you take it.

My colleague, Alan Gaby, M.D., stated the situation elegantly in his book, *B_6: The Natural Healer* (Keats Publishing, 1987): "We are grateful to modern medical science for what it has given us. Antibiotics, hormones, new surgical techniques, and advanced diagnostic devices have saved many lives. Yet, medicine as it is practiced today is too expensive, too dangerous, and too often ineffective. The evidence continues to mount that diet and nutrient therapy can be a safe, effective, and inexpensive alternative to drugs and surgery."

Potent Substances

Dietary supplements are potent substances. Microscopic amounts can prevent deficiency diseases, and larger amounts may be therapeutic for a wide variety of health problems. Some health problems are chronic, nagging symptoms that may be relieved temporarily by medicine, only to recur when your susceptibility is high. Common examples are allergies, eczema, headaches, hypoglycemia, digestive upset, anxiety, acne, fatigue, arthritis, sinusitis, and asthma (which may be more severe than the others). These illnesses are not usually lethal, but they can make your life miserable. Most medical therapies do not deal with them effectively or prevent their recurrence.

Other health problems are more serious. It is estimated that 85 percent of the chronic, degenerative diseases that kill people are related to lifestyle choices. These include heart disease, diabetes, cancer, hypertension, and stroke. The lifestyle choices that influence them are diet, smoking, alcohol, nontherapeutic drugs, caffeine consumption, exercise, dietary supplements, and stress reduction.

Dietary supplements have a strong effect on the development and relief of all of these uncomfortable or life-threatening problems. They can both relieve symptoms and prevent relapse. They can also reduce the incidence of and risk of dying from potentially lethal diseases such as heart disease, diabetes, and cancer. I have been saying this for twenty-five years, based on literature reports that were definitive or strongly suggestive, and on the long safety record of dietary supplements. The research support is even stronger now than when I started.

Prevention and Treatment

In the past few years, an increasing number of scientific studies have been confirming the view that nutrients are therapeutic and preventive. Vitamins C and E, beta-carotene, selenium, zinc, and magnesium are among the many nutrients that have been shown to contribute positively to health and longevity. Even the National Cancer Institute is looking more favorably on vitamin C these days, especially due to the work of Dr. Linus Pauling. I was surprised to see an article several years ago in the prestigious *New England Journal of Medicine,* written by researcher Dr. Mark Levine, on the biology and biochemistry of vitamin C, suggesting that the RDA might not be adequate for optimal health. This idea was revolutionary for the mainstream medical press. (For an explanation of the RDAs, see the inset on page 23.)

Vitamins are generally defined as complex organic substances that are essential in the diet because they are not manufactured in the body, yet they participate in physiological reactions. The definition is not quite precise, because some substances, such as vitamin D, are produced in the body, although not necessarily in adequate quantities. Also, the body produces vitamin A (which is thus not a true vitamin) from beta-carotene, which is called a provitamin (incorrectly, because it is essential and cannot be made in the body). Some substances are not exactly vitamins, but they are like vitamins because they are part of other nutrients, such as para-aminobenzoic acid (PABA), choline, and inositol.

I have been taking dietary supplements for thirty years. I take a wide variety of vitamins, minerals, amino acids, essential fatty acids, flavonoids, and herbs. I usually take large doses of the most protective nutrients (I will tell you more about what I take later). You, too, can be a part of this health revolution. Making informed choices about dietary supplements in combination with a healthy diet, exercise, and stress management will have a positive influence on your life.

In the next chapters, you will find an explanation of many of the health benefits of specific dietary supplements that I have found helpful in my holistic medical practice. Large doses of many of these substances have been shown to lower cholesterol, decrease blood pressure, enhance immunity and resistance to infection, decrease the risk of cancer, slow the aging process, increase energy and stamina, improve sugar regulation, and restore healthy gum tissue. They also reduce the incidence of birth defects and miscarriage. They can probably help you reduce your frequency of colds and other infections, decrease allergy symptoms, improve your energy, and enhance your general sense of well-being. As you will see, these are only some of the reasons to take many of these dietary supplements.

All the substances described as antioxidants or free-radical scavengers help to slow the aging process; reduce the risk of cancer and heart disease; decrease skin wrinkling due to sun exposure, smoking, or age; detoxify environmental pollutants including cigarette smoke; decrease the production of age pigment in the skin ("liver spots" or "age spots"); and protect you from the damaging effects of X rays and ultraviolet light. Supplements as well as rich nutritional food sources are essential to reduce your risk of degenerative diseases and give you the best chance of living a long and healthy life.

All comprehensive health programs require more than just dietary supplements. When I design health programs, I use a health and medical history, laboratory tests, and educated intuition based on many years of experience, scientific literature, and discussions with colleagues who also have years of experience using dietary supplements. (This is the way most medicine is practiced, whether based on medication, surgery, or other treatments, and whether conventional or not. It is the art of medicine.)

Supplements are not only useful in the prevention of illness and maintenance of a positive state of health; many of them are also valuable in the treatment of specific medical conditions. However, none of these descriptions of the clinical usefulness of supplements is meant to serve as a prescription or as medical treatment without consultation with a health practitioner. These are some of the clinical applications of nutrients that are reasonably well supported in the medical literature and have helped patients in my experience, but these specific combinations may not be appropriate for you.

A Note on the RDAs

The Recommended Dietary Allowances are established by the Food and Nutrition Board of the National Research Council, National Academy of Science. These nutrient levels are supposed to prevent deficiency diseases in most healthy people. Unfortunately, not only science but also the food industry, economic considerations, and politics have heavily influenced the values.

Many researchers question the value of the RDAs. They make the highly processed American food supply look more nutritious than it is, and they appear to be influenced by the food industry. The RDAs are *not* useful in establishing *optimal* health. You are at little risk of developing the deficiency diseases—pellagra, scurvy, or beriberi. Our modern problems are not deficiency diseases but degenerative diseases. Nutrients play an important role in preventing these conditions. The RDAs cannot be used in evaluating the therapeutic and preventive value of large doses of dietary supplements.

The sad truth is, if you look around, you will see many people who do manage to get the RDA levels of most nutrients, but they still go on to develop premature heart disease, cancer, arthritis, strokes, and diabetes. They have frequent viral infections (colds, the flu, herpes), they are overweight, and they lose their teeth to decay and gum disease. In terms of life expectancy, infant mortality, and health-care costs, Americans are not in the most favorable position in world statistics. Average Americans have a lower life expectancy than citizens of some third-world countries do.

In this regard, it is not good to be average—the average American will die prematurely of those chronic, degenerative diseases mentioned above. You can do many things to improve your health and reduce your risk of developing the health problems of the rest of the population. Taking dietary supplements is one of them. And it is an important one.

Nutrients and Herbs

There are many substances that are clinically useful in physiological approaches to health care and preventive medicine. They are sometimes referred to by the generic term "vitamins," but they include vitamins, minerals, amino acids, essential fatty acids, and natural hormones. As mentioned above, there are also conditionally essential nutrients (those that are necessary in some circumstances, such as coenzyme Q_{10}, L-carnitine, and L-arginine) and accessory food factors (such as flavonoids), which have physiological functions but are not essential in the diet as far as we know.

In addition to these nutrients, there are natural therapeutic herbs and plant extracts from various traditional healing cultures such as the Chinese, Indian, and Native American. Technically, because herbs usually contain substances that are not normally present in the body, they are not part of orthomolecular medicine, but they are usually helpful in the healing process and many of them have little or no known toxicity. It is impossible to include all therapeutic herbs here. I have included some of those that I have found most useful in my practice.

This is not a comprehensive list of all the therapeutic uses of the products described, but it is a summary of the most important health relationships that I have found in clinical practice over the last twenty-four years. It would be wise to consult a professional for individual advice, especially if you have unusual health or medical needs. It is also a good idea to do a lot of self-education. Don't forget to include diet, exercise, stress management, and personal development as part of your comprehensive health plan.

Multivitamin/Mineral Supplements

It makes supplement programs much easier if you start out with a high-quality multivitamin/mineral combination. In these descriptions of how to take individual supplements, the basic recommended amounts for many of them will usually be found in such a multi, and you will probably need to take from four to eight tablets per day to get those doses. Sometimes the amount in a high-potency, comprehensive multi is adequate for most health needs if you do not want to take too many pills, but usually a number of additional supplements will enhance your health program.

The multivitamin/mineral that I use in my practice is a comprehensive professional formulation. Many nutritionally oriented physicians will use comparable formulas, and there are similar ones available from both retail health food stores and mail-order sources. (See Appendix 2 for several sources.) The following content list is the total that you will find in six tablets (the daily recommendation) of this particular formula. For convenience, it is called "Basic Multiple" in the next chapters. Check if your multi has similar figures, and it will make supplementing your diet much easier. If yours is slightly different, it may be of only minor significance. Larger differences can easily be adjusted by changing the doses of the specific nutrients involved, adding other sources to make up the difference, or you can look for a comparable formula.

The formula for *six* daily tablets of the Basic Multiple:

Vitamin A	10,000	*IU*	*Zinc*	30	*mg*
Vitamin C	1,200	*mg*	*Selenium*	200	*mcg*
Beta-carotene	15,000	*IU*	*Chromium*	200	*mcg*
Vitamin D_3	400	*IU*	*Copper*	3	*mg*
Vitamin E (natural)	400	*IU*	*Manganese*	20	*mg*
Thiamine (B_1)	100	*mg*	*Molybdenum*	100	*mcg*
Riboflavin (B_2)	50	*mg*	*Potassium*	99	*mg*
Niacinamide (B_3)	150	*mg*	*Choline*	150	*mg*
Niacin (B_3)	40	*mg*	*Citrus bioflavonoids*	100	*mg*
Pyridoxine (B_6)	100	*mg*	*PABA*	50	*mg*
Folate (folic acid)	800	*mcg*	*Vanadium*	50	*mcg*
Vitamin B_{12}	100	*mcg*	*Boron*	3	*mg*
Biotin	300	*mcg*	*L- and N-acetyl-cysteine*	200	*mg*
Pantothenic acid	500	*mg*	*Methionine*	62.5	*mg*
Calcium	500	*mg*	*Glutamic HCl*	25	*mg*
Magnesium	500	*mg*	*Betaine HCl*	150	*mg*
Iodine	200	*mcg*			

This Basic Multiple formula has the right balance of major nutrients in the essential quantities for basic good health. Calcium-to-magnesium ratios may vary somewhat in multiples from different sources. There are several variations of this formula (such as with iron or without copper) for special needs. In order to meet your individual needs, any multi that you choose should have that flexibility. Adjustment of specific nutrient doses is easy with additional supplements, beyond what is contained in any one multiple.

Remember that these nutrients are meant to be in addition to what you will obtain from your diet.

Units and Measurements

It may help you to have some explanations of dosage terminology before I describe the individual nutrients. A kilogram (kg) is a metric measure of weight equivalent to approximately 2.2 pounds, while a gram (g) is 1/1000 of a kilogram. A milligram (mg) is 1/1000 of a gram, and a microgram (mcg) is 1/1000 of a milligram, or one millionth of a gram.

International Units, or IU, are different for each nutrient. For example, for vitamin E they are determined with reference to biological activity in maintaining pregnancy in rats. One *milli*gram is approximately 1.49 IU of natural vitamin E. For vitamin A, International Units are measured in "retinol equivalents," and 1 *micro*gram is approximately 5 IU.

It is important not to make a mistake when reading units and weights, both for safety and for being sure you are getting what you are paying for. Read labels carefully and review this information, if necessary.

Nutrient Classifications

One way of classifying vitamins is by whether they are fat soluble or water soluble. The fat-soluble vitamins are vitamin A, carotenoids, and vitamins D, E, and K. Coenzyme Q_{10} is another fat-soluble nutrient, although it is not, strictly speaking, a vitamin. Essential fatty acids are obviously fat soluble, but they are worthy of their own discussion. Certain substances, such as mineral oil, some medications, and excesses of certain dietary substances may reduce the absorption of fat-soluble nutrients or some minerals.

One property of some of the fat-soluble nutrients is that they may be readily stored either in fatty tissue or in the liver. Vitamins A and D are known to have some toxicity as a result of accumulation of large amounts, so you need to be somewhat careful of the doses that you take. It is common for the general press and supplement antagonists to exaggerate the toxicity of these nutrients, but the usual doses are quite safe. If you take very large doses for prolonged periods, you do put yourself at some risk. The usual side effects are readily reversible, but some calcifications that can result from excess vitamin D may not be.

In spite of their being fat soluble, vitamin E and coenzyme Q_{10} are not stored excessively, and they are readily used up in performing their protective roles. There is no known toxicity from these nutrients at any of the doses that have been studied. Beta-carotene is also nontoxic, although with high doses or high dietary amounts your skin may take on a harmless orange-yellow hue known as carotenemia.

The B vitamins and vitamin C are water soluble. Water-soluble nutrients have a reputation of being quite safe in almost any doses because they are not stored in the body (except for vitamin B_{12}, which is stored in the liver but is still not toxic). For the most part, any excess intake is readily excreted in the urine. This reputation for safety is *almost* entirely deserved, but not quite. There are a few problems from excessive doses of vitamin B_3 (niacin), especially in the timed-release form, and vitamin B_6 (pyridoxine). The doses required for such side effects are usually enormous compared with typical therapeutic levels. The side effects have usually been completely reversible. It is wise to be aware of these risks but not overly anxious about them. Most of the problems are minor, but occasionally some are more serious. They are discussed under the description of each nutrient.

The minerals, amino acids, accessory food factors, and flavonoids are not generally classified according to solubility. There are also many therapeutic herbs/botanicals and some miscellaneous substances that are valuable in health care. At the end of each supplement description, there is a brief explanation of how to take it, and in what forms it is most conveniently available.

If you have significant health problems, you need to be aware of the value of good professional medical care, and you should seek such advice. If you can find a physician in your area who understands nutritional therapy and might use it instead of medication, so much the better. If not, perhaps you can introduce your physician to these concepts. (See Appendix 2 for ways to find nutritionally oriented physicians.)

The explanation of dietary supplements in this book is meant to be brief, but it should give you enough information to know what supplements to take and in what amounts for general good health and vitality. It is not a textbook or a research paper, and it is not a medical prescription. However, you will find some references and other resources if you want to pursue further information.

Now, on to the supplements.

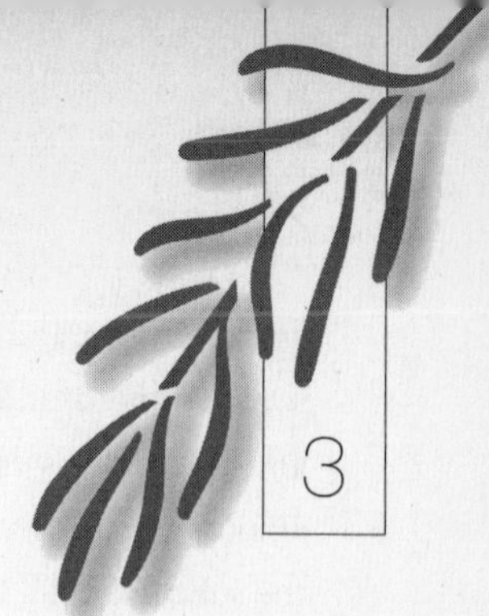

Fat-Soluble Nutrients

As mentioned in the previous chapter, fat-soluble nutrients are those that are stored in the fatty tissues of the body. They are more likely to accumulate in these tissues, and occasionally they can cause problems if you take too many.

Carotenes

Beta-carotene and alpha-carotene are two of a group of nutrients called carotenoids, which also includes lycopene, zeaxanthin, and others that provide some of the color in green, yellow, and orange fruits and vegetables. Carotenoids are highly effective antioxidants, even in tissues where oxygen levels are low (other antioxidants don't work as well in tissues with low oxygen levels). Some of the beta-carotene is converted in the body into vitamin A, and although both are antioxidant, beta-carotene is more active. The body has a feedback mechanism that protects it from excess conversion into vitamin A, so that you have no worries about toxicity from carotenoids.

A large body of scientific research shows that carotenoids help protect against cancer and heart disease and the degeneration from free radicals. In some animal studies, they have even led to the regression of some cancers, and in humans to regression of some precancerous conditions. High amounts of carotenoids as supplements or from food can lead to deposits in the subcutaneous fat and make your skin appear orange. This is a harmless condition known as carotenemia. In fact, this slightly yellow-orange skin color is a good sign, indicating that you have some extra protection from the powerful oxygen-generated free radicals. Lutein has recently become available as a supplement (6 to 20 mg) that helps prevent macular degeneration, a deterioration with age of the most sensitive area of the retina. Lycopene is another carotene that may help with macular degeneration and in the prevention and treatment of prostate cancer.

The most common carotenoid supplement is beta-carotene, but mixed carotenoids from natural sources are probably better. This is often called simply natural beta-carotene. Recent studies have suggested that taking synthetic beta-carotene by itself as a supplement may increase cancer risk in heavy smokers, although those subjects who had high levels of beta-carotene from their diets appeared to have a lower risk. This emphasizes the importance of following a healthy diet, and not depending solely on supplements for your nutrition. Natural mixed carotenoids are available as a supplement (it will say derived from *D. salina* on the label). Most multivitamins contain the synthetic beta-carotene as it is more stable.

How to Take Carotenoids Carotenoids are usually available as 25,000-IU capsules. Look for the natural carotenoids, although they are more expensive than the synthetic. I suggest 25,000 IU in addition to the 15,000 that is in Basic Multiple, and for cancer patients and people exposed to high levels of carcinogens (such as secondhand smoke) I often recommend even more, taken in balance with other antioxidants. Lycopene is available separately in 5 to 10 mg capsules, and lutein is available in 10 to 20 mg capsules.

Vitamin A

This vitamin helps you to maintain the quality of your mucous membranes and to resist infections. Vitamin A is essential for normal vision, bone growth, reproduction, and white blood cell development. It is also essential for normal immune function and fertility. It is found naturally only in animal products, but it can be made by the body from beta-carotene. The conversion from beta-carotene is an enzymatic reaction in the intestines, and this process may be sluggish. Therefore, in certain situations, it may be beneficial to take the preformed vitamin A, instead of depending on the conversion. It helps to protect the membranes from the effects of pollutants such as cigarette smoke and car exhaust. It is also useful in skin conditions such as acne. Vitamin A has some activity as an antioxidant, but not as much as beta-carotene.

Although large doses of vitamin A are potentially toxic, there is a fairly wide margin of safety in adults. However, I recommend that you avoid taking very large doses (over 50,000 to 100,000 IU) without first consulting your health practitioner. Avoid doses above 10,000 IU during the first three months of pregnancy. Sometimes the larger doses are used therapeutically for a short time, and some physicians use massive doses for cancer patients.

How to Take Vitamin A Vitamin A is commonly available in 10,000- and 25,000-IU capsules and in multivitamins. The Basic Multiple formula contains 10,000 IU. When I recommend extra, I usually suggest one capsule of 25,000 IU. I then adjust the dose depending on the clinical situation.

Vitamin D

Vitamin D is produced in the body (and therefore it is not a true vitamin) by the action of ultraviolet light from the sun on the cholesterol in the skin. For this reason it has been called the "sunshine" vitamin, but it is really more a steroid hormone than a vitamin. As we age, our ability to produce vitamin D in the skin declines, and our ability to absorb it is reduced. In addition, it is common for older people to have less exposure to the sun and poorer intestinal absorption, so they may need more supplements of vitamin D.

Vitamin D_3 (cholecalciferol, the natural form of vitamin D) is required for normal calcium absorption, balance, and utilization. It works with parathyroid hormone to maintain normal blood levels of calcium. It is essential for bone formation and maintenance and for those nerve and cell functions that depend on calcium.

The conversion of vitamin D to its more active metabolites takes place in the kidneys. In liver or kidney impairment, or bowel disorders, supplements of vitamin D may be necessary. Although dairy products contain added vitamin D, it is the synthetic form, or vitamin D_2 (irradiated ergosterol), that is usually used.

High levels of vitamin D are potentially toxic, leading to excessive calcification of the tissues. People consuming a lot of dairy products, other commercial animal products, and processed fortified foods (none of which I recommend) may get more than enough vitamin D. The tissue calcifications from excess vitamin D are often irreversible. It is therefore important to be careful about overdoing supplements, especially if you are unwilling to eliminate processed foods and excessive animal products from your diet. Excess vitamin D may lead to calcium accumulation inside cells as we age, interfering with enzyme activity and increasing the degenerative diseases of aging. However; moderate supplements of vitamin D, especially for the elderly, are valuable to maintain proper calcium balance.

How to Take Vitamin D The Basic Multiple formula (and many common multis on the market) contains 400 IU of vitamin D. I usually do not use more than this amount, although in some elderly patients an extra 400 IU may be beneficial. Supplement capsules with 400 IU are available, usually mixed with vitamin A. Fish liver oils are another common source of vitamin D supplements. They are available as liquids or capsules, and they vary in their A and D content.

Vitamin E

Natural vitamin E (as *d*-alpha tocopherol plus the mixed tocopherols—beta, gamma, and delta) is a good biological antioxidant, protecting you from the ravages of free-radical pathology, heart disease, cancer, and aging. Synthetic vitamin E (*dl*-alpha) is about 50 percent less active than the natural form. Be careful when reading the label, as that little *l* after the *d* may be obscure. The forms other than alpha are not used to characterize the potency of the capsules of vitamin E, but they are active, and the gamma form may be at least as important as the alpha. I, myself, take a vitamin E with increased levels of the mixed tocopherols.

Vitamin E is found naturally in plant oils, such as seeds, nuts and grains, and also in some green vegetables. Almonds are a particularly rich source, but in order to get the healthiest amounts of vitamin E it would be necessary to eat too much fat in the diet. Although vitamin E is found in natural vegetable oils, commercial processing (solvent extraction, filtering, bleaching, and deodorizing) eliminates much of the vitamin from the end product. Extra polyunsaturated oil in the diet (not a good idea) increases the need for vitamin E, which protects the unsaturated fatty acids from oxidation. Poor fat digestion or absorption can reduce the amount of vitamin E that actually gets into your bloodstream from foods.

Vitamin E helps maintain healthy circulation in the coronary arteries and peripheral blood vessels. In fact, blood levels of vitamin E are more than twice as predictive of heart disease risk as cholesterol levels (high levels of vitamin E mean a lower incidence of heart disease). It can relieve exercise-induced leg or heart pain by improving the efficiency of oxygen use. Vitamin E decreases platelet stickiness, which reduces excessive blood clotting, thereby offering protection from thrombosis, or sudden blockage of an artery. It can also lower total blood cholesterol levels, while it helps to raise the good cholesterol known as HDL (high-density lipoprotein). In the oxidized state, the so-called bad cholesterol, or LDL (low-density lipoprotein), is damaging to the arterial lining, and vitamin E can prevent the oxidation of this LDL, thereby protecting arteries from atherosclerosis.

It can help with leg cramps including those that occur at night, and also with premenstrual cramps. In many women, vitamin E can reverse fibrocystic breast disease (but you may also need to give up all caffeine if this is your problem).

Doses of 200 to 800 IU per day of vitamin E enhance immune function in the elderly by increasing the activity of the white blood cells (which destroy viruses and bacteria as well as stray cancer cells) and by increasing antibody production. This leads to higher resistance and results in fewer infections. This is particularly important since the elderly are frequently more susceptible to infections. Vitamin E can also relieve menopausal hot flashes, although sometimes fairly high doses are necessary, up to 1,200 or even 2,000 IU.

Tocopherols are necessary for normal neurologic function, and they protect against environmental toxins and peroxidation of the lipids (fats) in cell membranes. (Peroxidation is the addition of excess oxygen to molecules and is the same process responsible for rancidity of foods.) This peroxidation leads to the formation of free radicals, which hasten the aging process and cause damage to the skin and blood vessels.

As an antioxidant, vitamin E works intimately with other antioxidants and free-radical scavengers such as selenium, glutathione, carotenoids, and vitamin C. This is one example of how nutrients work synergistically to have effects that are greater than those obtained when the substances are taken separately. Vitamin E also protects dietary essential fatty acids from oxidation.

How to Take Vitamin E The usual preventive and therapeutic doses that I use range from 400 to 1,200 IU per day, but in some cases patients may need 2,000 IU or more. There is no known toxicity at these doses, although high doses of vitamin E can enhance the activity of coumadin, the anticlotting drug. This is easy for physicians to monitor, as they measure the effects of coumadin regularly, and can just lower the coumadin dose, if necessary. I always give patients 400 IU in the Basic Multiple and usually an additional 400 IU or 800 IU if they are elderly or have blood vessel diseases.

For menopausal hot flashes I sometimes recommend up to 2,000 IU per day, but with proper diet, other nutrient supplements and hormonal balance, such high doses are not usually needed. Herbs for menopause, such as Dong quai, black cohosh, and Vitex agnus castus, may reduce the need for high doses of vitamin E. It is not possible, from diet alone, to consume adequate amounts of vitamin E for optimal health. For the full protection vitamin E has to offer, you must take supplements.

Vitamin K

Although I have not used vitamin K as a supplement, some of my colleagues do, and it is worth mentioning. It occurs naturally in two fat-soluble forms—phylloquinone, from plants (leafy green vegetables), and menaquinone, produced by your own friendly intestinal bacteria. Natural vitamin K is virtually nontoxic. (Menadione is a water-soluble synthetic substitute, and it does have potential toxic effects.)

Vitamin K is essential for normal blood clotting and normal bone formation. Deficiency is not usually a problem because of intestinal bacterial production. However, with various bowel diseases there may be inadequate production, and with fat malabsorption, dietary sources may be inadequately absorbed. With antibiotic therapy, the intestinal bacterial source may be reduced to zero, and supplements of friendly bacteria can help restore normal vitamin K production.

There are a few possible therapeutic uses for a supplement of vitamin K, but so far the therapeutic doses are mainly available by prescription, although smaller doses are found in some multivitamin preparations. In deficiencies that result from bowel inflammation or antibiotic treatment, vitamin K can restore normal blood clotting. For patients taking anticlotting medications, taking vitamin K can interfere with the actions of the medication. Do not take vitamin K supplements without medical advice in these situations. When administered with extra vitamin C, it can relieve morning sickness in pregnancy, at a dose of 5 mg per day. Finally, it may help relieve inflammation and arthritis and improve bone density.

How to Take Vitamin K For higher doses of vitamin K, you will need to see a nutritionally oriented physician. Smaller amounts are available in combinations containing 80–100 mcg, a variable dose taken once or twice per day.

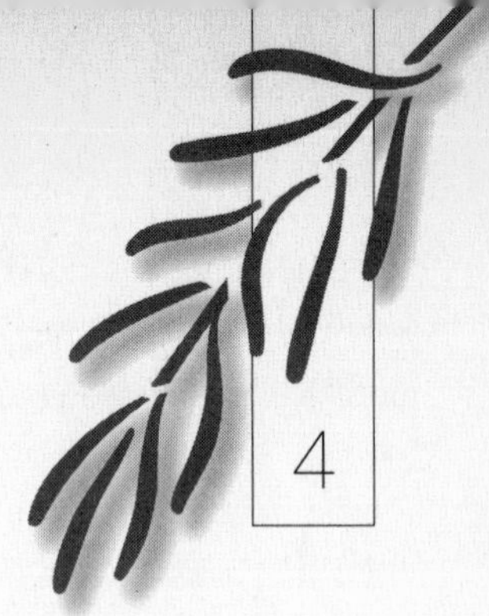

4

Water-Soluble Nutrients

WATER-SOLUBLE VITAMINS include the B complex vitamins and vitamin C. They are readily absorbed through the intestinal lining and easily excreted through the kidneys. Any extra that you consume is usually simply excreted, and they have very little risk of toxicity. While B_{12} has special requirements for absorption, if you take enough, it will be absorbed by simple diffusion even in the absence of those other factors.

B-Complex Vitamins

There are quite a few B vitamins. Most are numbered (thiamine = B_1; riboflavin = B_2; niacin or niacinamide = B_3; pantothenic acid = B_5; pyridoxine = B_6; and cobalamin = B_{12}), but folic acid is not. Several other nutrients considered part of the B complex include choline, inositol, biotin, lipoic acid, para-aminobenzoic acid, and dimethyl glycine. The B vitamins have a variety of functions, and they frequently work together. It was thought at one time that you had to take equal amounts of all the B vitamins to be balanced. This is not quite true, since some people need different amounts of each one for their particular metabolism, and high doses of individual B vitamins may be therapeutic for specific conditions.

Examples of the therapeutic use of B complex vitamins include the treatment of carpal tunnel syndrome and PMS with pyridoxine (B_6), and the treatment of mental illness and high cholesterol with niacin (B_3). You might be interested to know that this treatment of high cholesterol with high doses of niacin is one of the few orthomolecular treatments accepted by orthodox medicine (of course, they don't call it orthomolecular).

Having regular injections of vitamin B_{12} is the usual treatment for pernicious anemia (anemia due to poor absorption of the vitamin), because of the requirements for hydrochloric acid, a substance called "intrinsic factor," and a healthy intestinal lining to absorb it. Even without these factors, however, a high enough oral dose can be absorbed by simple diffusion, thus making injections unnecessary. High does of vitamin B_{12} can help many patients with fatigue and depression, even when a deficiency cannot be demonstrated. Vitamin B_{12} is one of the supplements that can lower homocysteine levels, and thus reduce the risk of developing heart disease (also see the discussion of pyridoxine, on page 41), and it can help with osteoarthritis.

Vitamin B_2 (riboflavin) is important for the maintenance of adequate antioxidant enzyme levels. It helps with cataract prevention, muscle cramps, and immune function. I usually suggest only the 50 mg that is in the Basic Multiple. Recent evidence shows that 400 mg per day can reduce the frequency and severity of migraine headaches. It is riboflavin that gives the urine its intense yellow color when any leftover is excreted. This is a harmless effect.

Thiamine (Vitamin B_1)

Thiamine is a water-soluble vitamin essential in energy metabolism (normal oxidation). Marginal deficiencies of thiamine are quite common, usually related to the overconsumption of refined foods, including white flour and sugar, which displace nutrient-rich whole foods in the diet. Symptoms of deficiency include numbness and tingling of the extremities, generalized musculoskeletal tenderness (similar to some of the symptoms of fibromyalgia), heart problems, palpitations, and a variety of neuropsychological ailments, including hyperawareness of abnormal bodily functions. Low blood pressure and dizziness are also possible signs of inadequate thiamine.

Dr. Derrick Lonsdale, a preventive medicine physician and researcher, has studied these symptoms of low thiamine and calls them "functional dysautonomia." This refers to abnormalities of the autonomic nervous system (the part you don't usually control but you can influence), which controls background physiological functions such as temperature, blood pressure, heart rate, glandular secretions, sweating, and intestinal and bladder functions. His research suggests that large doses of thiamine (up to 600 mg daily) may be necessary to correct some of these symptoms.

How to Take Thiamine Supplements of 50 to 500 mg of thiamine are often clinically useful. I usually suggest only 100 mg, the amount that is in the Basic Multiple, but on occasion I have suggested more. Another form, much less common but helpful for some people with dysautonomia is allithiamin, which is a fat-soluble form that is more active than plain thiamine.

Niacin and Niacinamide (Vitamin B_3)

Niacin is another important B-complex vitamin. It was formerly called nicotinic acid, but the name was changed because it was confused with nicotine by some people. Niacin supplements lower total cholesterol and raise the good (HDL) cholesterol. It was the first nutrient used in the "megavitamin" treatment of mental disorders, by Drs. Hoffer and Osmond in the early 1950s. In my clinical experience, the timed-release form of niacin helps to minimize hypoglycemic symptoms, especially during withdrawal from sugar. It usually reduces cravings for sweets. In many patients, high doses help with depression.

Because niacin can dilate blood vessels, it can lower blood pressure and also improve circulation. It can reduce migraine headaches and Raynaud's phenomenon. The latter is a circulation disorder with spasms of the arteries in the hands when exposed to cold. Many patients who suffer from Ménière's disease, with vertigo or dizzy spells, find relief with niacin supplements. Niacin is one of the nutrients in an orthomolecular program used for the management of drug and alcohol addiction during the withdrawal period.

Plain and sometimes even timed-release niacin can cause a flush of the skin that feels like an allergic reaction. This is the result of a histamine release similar to what happens with an allergy, and it usually disappears within fifteen to twenty minutes. If you take niacin regularly, the flush usually stops happening because the histamine levels in the tissues are constantly drained. This flush is usually reduced or eliminated with the timed-release form of niacin, which I have used safely in many patients for years. However, the timed-release niacin can sometimes cause elevation of liver enzymes and, on rare occasions, has caused hepatitis in sensitive individuals.

Do not take niacin, either plain or timed release, if you have active peptic ulcer disease or gout (arthritis due to uric acid deposits), since it can increase uric acid levels and gastric acid production. A different form of niacin, inositol hexaniacinate, has several advantages: it causes no flush and has the same cholesterol-lowering capacity as regular niacin. It has never been shown to cause liver problems. The inositol hexaniacinate form does not cause uric acid elevation or histamine-induced gastric acid release and is therefore not a problem in gout or ulcer disease.

Niacinamide is another molecular form of vitamin B_3. It does not cause a flush because it does not release histamine, but it also does not lower cholesterol. It does help arthritis, insomnia, and anxiety for many patients, but it does not help Ménière's, migraines, or Raynaud's phenomenon. Without a histamine release, it is not a problem in gout or ulcer disease.

How to Take Niacin and Niacinamide The Basic Multiple formula contains 150 mg of niacinamide and 40 mg of niacin (an amount unlikely to cause a flush because the dose is divided, although it may in some sensitive people). Niacin is available as 250- to 500-mg timed-release tablets, and inositol hexaniacinate is available as 400- to 500-mg capsules. Therapeutic doses of niacin range from 250 mg twice per day up to 1,000 mg three times per day. I often suggest 400 to 800 mg of inositol hexaniacinate twice per day for patients with elevated cholesterol. For hypoglycemics, I often start them on the timed-release form, 250 mg twice per day.

Niacinamide doses are the same as for niacin in managing arthritis and psychiatric disorders.For arthritis, the effective daily dose of niacinamide is between 2,000 and 3,000 mg to start. These can be reduced to 1,000 to 1,500 mg after the symptoms are relieved. It is available as 500-mg capsules or tablets.

Pantothenic Acid and Pantethine (Vitamin B_5)

Pantothenic acid was discovered by Dr. Roger Williams, the originator of the concept of biochemical individuality. This vitamin is essential for the adrenal glands to produce their hormones. The adrenal glands help maintain us in times of stress, during which these glands can become exhausted and unable to respond to stress by producing adequate hormones. They need extra pantothenic acid (as well as vitamin C) to restore their normal function.

A deficiency of pantothenic acid can lead to depression, fatigue, and insomnia. Requirements for pantothenic acid are higher during pregnancy and lactation. Some physicians are also using high doses for inflammatory arthritis. I often recommend high doses of pantothenic acid for my patients with recurrent illnesses, environmental toxicity, allergies, or high stress levels.The coenzyme form of pantothenic acid is called pantethine. When taken as a supplement, most of it appears to be converted to pantothenic acid before absorption. However, unlike plain pantothenic acid, this coenzyme form can help lower total cholesterol and triglyceride levels, and raise the good HDL-cholesterol levels.

How to Take Panthothenic Acid Pantothenic acid is generally sold as calcium pantothenate and it is commonly available in 500-mg tablets or capsules, which contain a little bit of calcium in addition to the pantothenate. I usually recommend 500 mg per day as part of Basic Multiple. I may suggest up to 2,000 mg to those patients experiencing very high stress levels. For pantethine, a daily dose of 900 mg is usually adequate for the benefits to cholesterol and triglyceride levels. It is available in 300 to 500 mg capsules. I often recommend 500 mg twice per day.

PYRIDOXINE (VITAMIN B_6)

Pyridoxine was another discovery of Dr. Albert Szent-Györgyi, in 1938. This vitamin is necessary for antibody formation, enzyme activity, smooth muscle function, and fatty acid metabolism. It is a cofactor for many enzymes. (Cofactors are those elements or molecules required for enzyme activity.) Deficiencies of vitamin B_6 can lead to anemia, dermatitis, and neuropathy. The dermatitis associated with B_6 deficiency is easily mistaken for essential fatty acid deficiency, and it is common for fatty acid deficiency to occur at the same time as increased need for pyridoxine.

Pyridoxine supplements have helped women who have nausea and vomiting during pregnancy, or "morning sickness," and, combined with magnesium, have reduced symptoms of pre-eclampsia—signs of this condition (also called toxemia of pregnancy) are fluid retention, high blood pressure, and protein leaking into the urine; if severe, it can lead to convulsions. B_6 also reduces birth defects. It has been used to treat PMS, depression, childhood autism, and asthma. (For asthma, B_6 works better when combined with magnesium, vitamin C, and some essential fatty acids.)

B_6 has also helped to reduce the incidence of the common oxalate type of kidney stones, particularly when taken with magnesium. You can also prevent headaches related to MSG in the "Chinese restaurant syndrome" if you take enough B_6 in advance. Of course, it is better to avoid the MSG in the first place (it is used in other kinds of restaurants also).

There is a significantly increased risk of heart disease in people with high blood levels of a metabolite called homocysteine. Serum levels of homocysteine may be more significant than cholesterol levels in predicting the risk of heart disease. Your homocysteine level is likely to be increased if you do not have enough of the vitamins B_6, B_{12}, folic acid, and betaine (derived from choline). Supplements of these nutrients have been shown to reduce homocysteine levels. (This work, originally by Kilmer McCully, M.D., is thirty years old but was rejected by the medical community until recently.)

Pyridoxine supplements have been helpful in the treatment of peripheral neuropathy (nerve damage to the extremities with numbness, tingling and a "pins-and-needles" sensation), but some reports have shown a relationship of very high doses of B_6 to the *development* of neuropathy, if taken for many months. The doses that have been harmful were from 2,000 to 6,000 mg per day, far above the recommended levels for therapeutic supplementation, but it should be used with caution. Isolated reports suggested similar adverse effects with doses as low as 500 mg, but these reports have not been confirmed. Many women have taken this level for treatment of premenstrual syndrome (PMS). No confirmed reports show a risk of toxicity with less than 500 mg.

How to Take Pyridoxine I usually recommend the 100 mg that is in Basic Multiple, but some multis have reduced the dose of B_6 because of the reports of neuropathy from very high doses. I still think that 100 mg is quite safe. Additional B_6 is available as 100-, 250- and 500-mg capsules or tablets. I usually suggest an additional 250 mg for PMS and carpal tunnel syndrome. B_6 may lead to intense dreams and restless sleep when taken at night. It is best to take any extra doses with breakfast.

Folic Acid

Folic acid is found largely in "foliage," or green leafy vegetables, from which it gets its name. Also called folate or folacin, this B vitamin is especially important before and during pregnancy. It is necessary for the health of the fetus, preventing neural tube birth defects, such as spina bifida (incomplete closure of the spine). It has been estimated that 75 percent of such birth defects could be prevented with folic acid supplements. This information has been known for well over twenty-five years, but the FDA is only recently allowing such health claims for folic acid. And, even though the birth defect studies were done with supplements, the FDA insists that any label claims on supplements must say it is better to get the folate from food (asking the supplement company to say on their own label that it is better not to take the supplement!).

Folic acid is important in protection from cancer. It is beneficial for reversing cervical dysplasia, which are the precursor cells to cervical cancer seen on abnormal Pap smears. Folic acid is also helpful in preventing lung cancer. It has also been shown to lower blood levels of homocysteine, lowering your risk of heart disease (also see the discussion of pyridoxine, above).

Folate is also useful for the prevention and treatment of gum disease, the most common cause of tooth loss. It has this protective effect when applied topically to the gums. Unfortunately, folic acid has a reputation for causing vitamin B_{12} deficiency. This is *not* the case. High doses may *mask* the early signs of B_{12}-deficiency anemia (seen in a microscopic evaluation of the blood), making it somewhat more difficult to detect, but they do not cause it.

With currently available tests for adequacy of B_{12}, the detection of B_{12}-deficiency anemia is not dependent on the blood smear. However, the FDA limitation on the sale of high-dose folic acid remains in effect, ostensibly to protect the consumer. In reality, there is no reason to protect people from something that is harmless.

The maximum over-the-counter dose of folate is 800 mcg (0.8 mg). To get high doses, you have to take multiple pills, or see a physician who can prescribe higher doses. I often recommend daily doses of 5 mg for women planning pregnancy, or as early in pregnancy as possible. Recent evidence suggests that this same dose plus 1,000 mcg of vitamin B_{12} will benefit people with osteoarthritis of the hands, and it is very likely that this would also help arthritis of other joints.

Another use of high-dose folic acid is the prevention and treatment of gout. A metabolite of folate, commonly present in supplements, blocks the activity of xanthine oxidase, an enzyme that leads to the production of uric acid. This is the substance that is deposited in the joints in gout, or in the urinary tract, causing kidney stones. For patients with high uric acid, massive doses, up to 80 mg or more, may be helpful, although the research is unclear. With a comprehensive health program, including a proper diet, doses of 20 mg may be a worthwhile addition in the treatment of gout.

How to Take Folic Acid In the United States, folic acid is only available in high doses by prescription, and many nutritionally oriented doctors will prescribe it in 5- to 20-mg capsules. If you want to take preventive doses without a doctor's prescription, you need to get 800-mcg tablets and take several per day, for a total daily dose up to 5 mg. The Basic Multiple contains 800 mcg.

Vitamin B_{12} (Cobalamin)

Vitamin B_{12} is unlike the other water-soluble vitamins in that it is stored in the liver, making signs of any deficiency very slow to appear (up to five or six years with no intake before it is detected). In spite of its storage, it is not known to be toxic. The main dietary source is animal products, such as fish and eggs, with smaller amounts in milk and meat, so vegetarians should take a supplement. Although it is not well absorbed from the intestinal tract, especially in elderly people, if you take high-enough doses as a supplement enough can be absorbed to be therapeutic.

B_{12} is important for blood formation, nerve function, maintaining low levels of homocysteine to protect from heart disease and stroke, and maintaining mood and energy in elderly people. The required amount is very small, only about two micrograms per day, but you need to take a large amount to absorb that dose.

How to take Vitamin B_{12} I recommend 1,000 to 2,000 mcg of vitamin B_{12} for strict vegetarians or for patients with high homocysteine levels, or diabetic neuropathy, and for elderly patients with fatigue, depression, or Alzheimer's disease. It is usually available as 1,000-mcg sublingual tablets, although you do not have to dissolve them in the mouth for the benefits.

Other B Vitamins

There are therapeutic and preventive values for the other substances often considered part of the B complex. Large doses of *para-aminobenzoic acid* (PABA) are helpful in a sclerosing penile disorder called Peyronie's disease.

Dimethyl glycine (DMG) has been called pangamic acid and vitamin B_{15} in the past, but it is not a true vitamin. It may help to enhance immunity and improve the utilization of oxygen at the tissue level, and early studies suggested it could enhance endurance in athletes. Some colleagues have found it helpful in some cases of autism. I often recommend 125 mg dissolved in the mouth three or four times per day. DMG is an interesting substance in that it is "hygroscopic," meaning it absorbs water from the atmosphere. If left to sit out in the air, it will absorb enough water to dissolve itself. It is therefore packaged in individually wrapped, sealed foil packets.

Choline, a component of lecithin, is manufactured in the body and is a part of the neurotransmitter acetylcholine. It has been shown to significantly affect brain function when taken as a supplement. Large doses are helpful in tardive dyskinesia (awkward, uncontrollable facial and body movements), a condition that results from long-term use of antipsychotic medications called phenothiazines, including Thorazine, Stelazine, Mellaril, Prolixin, and others.

Inositol is also found in lecithin. Both inositol and choline are important for fatty acid transport, and they have a reputation for lowering cholesterol levels in the blood. However, research shows a number of other dietary supplements to be more effective for lowering cholesterol. Some people find inositol supplements beneficial for anxiety and insomnia.

Choline and inositol are not strictly water soluble but are more like emulsifiers. Because they have properties of both fat and water solubility, and because of their metabolic properties, they are known as "lipotropic" agents.

Both choline and inositol are part of compounds known as phospholipids, which are highly concentrated in nervous tissue. Phosphatidyl choline and phosphatidyl inositol are components of lecithins, found in egg yolks and legumes, especially soybeans. Another phospholipid, phosphatidylserine, is not considered a vitamin, and it is described in the chapter on accessory supplements.

Vitamin C

Vitamin C, technically ascorbic acid or ascorbate, is one of the most important nutrients. It is also one of the most remarkable substances in biology, having unique effects on the basic properties of molecules, cells, and tissues. Most animals make their own vitamin C, and they can make huge amounts (especially compared with the RDA!). A goat, for example, can make 13,000 mg of vitamin C in one day, and more if it is under stress.

Ascorbic acid gets its name from the fact that it cures scurvy. It has been known for over four hundred years that citrus fruits cure scurvy, but it took more than two hundred years and another scientific study before the British navy routinely provided this easy cure to its sailors. (The study by James Lind that led to this change was done on only nine sailors, but the results could not have been better, even if it had been a large-scale, double-blind, placebo-controlled trial. No responsible professional in this field is at all opposed to such necessary research studies, but we recognize that there are also other ways to acquire knowledge.) It is from this practice of providing citrus fruit to the navy that, even to this day, British people are called "limeys." Albert Szent-Györgyi discovered and extracted the active substance from fruits and vegetables in the 1920s.

Linus Pauling subsequently collaborated with Dr. Ewan Cameron on a study showing benefits to cancer patients from vitamin C in doses of 10 g per day. Their patients had fewer symptoms and greater longevity with supplements, compared with matched controls. Pauling and Cameron wrote a book about this, *Cancer and Vitamin C*. The National Cancer Institute only recently began taking this important information seriously.

Vitamin C has a wide range of metabolic functions. It is an excellent biological antioxidant, offering protection from oxidative free-radical damage. It is essential for the production of collagen, which is the connective tissue that holds us together. Without adequate collagen production, we would literally fall apart. In fact, the early symptoms of scurvy, easy bruising and bleeding gums, which are the signs of deteriorating connective tissue, are the results of poor collagen production.

As a consequence of both its role in collagen strength and its antioxidant activity, vitamin C reduces the wrinkling and sagging of the skin that occurs with aging. Vitamin C also helps maintain mucous membranes, and it is essential for the production of the adrenal gland hormones, which are readily depleted in times of stress.

Vitamin C promotes immune function, partly by enhancing interferon production. Interferon is the natural antiviral substance that your cells produce when you are infected with a virus. Interferon is now available as a very expensive medication, but one of the best ways to increase your interferon is to take supplements of vitamin C.

Ascorbic acid also helps immunity by increasing two different activities of your white blood cells. Some varieties of these cells produce protective antibodies (humoral immunity) and other white cells eat stray cancer cells, bacteria, and viruses (cellular immunity—not appetizing, but it can keep you healthy). Vitamin C promotes both of these functions and also helps to detoxify environmental pollutants.

It is interesting that during an infection, the level of vitamin C in the white blood cells drops precipitously. This is just when they need it the most! When supplements of 200 mg per day are administered, very little happens to the ascorbate level in the cells. Only when 6,000 mg per day are given does the level stay above normal, giving the cells a better chance to fight the infection.

In addition to enhancing interferon production, ascorbate also has its own antiviral properties, having been shown to kill some viruses if the tissue concentration is high enough. This is probably the basis for the successful use of intravenous vitamin C for viral illnesses such as hepatitis, mononucleosis, and influenza. Even taken orally in adequate doses, vitamin C reduces the symptoms of colds and other infections, including hepatitis, mononucleosis, and flu. Giving high doses of ascorbate intravenously is often necessary to adequately raise tissue levels for the treatment of infections.

Large oral doses, even up to 20 to 30 g or more, or intravenous treatment with vitamin C, can help with chronic fatigue syndrome, autoimmune disorders, multiple or severe allergies, and asthma. Asthma patients can increase their exercise tolerance by taking vitamin C before beginning exercise. Usually, 1 g taken about a half hour before exercise reduces or eliminates wheezing.

Ascorbate also helps with environmental illness related to exposure to toxic chemicals. Some patients with "Gulf War syndrome" have benefited from high oral and intravenous doses of vitamin C (along with other supplements). Gulf War syndrome is characterized by symptoms including fatigue, muscle and joint pain, inability to concentrate, headache, impaired memory, sleep disturbances, agitation, and respiratory symptoms, very much like chronic fatigue and multiple chemical sensitivity syndromes. Vitamin C protects the lining cells of the arteries, called endothelium, which produce nitric oxide. Nitric oxide helps to relax the blood vessel muscles and improve blood flow and blood pressure (see the discussion of L-arginine).

If you take too much vitamin C, the only potential side effect is slightly loose bowels or even diarrhea, an indication that you need to reduce the dose a little. Actually, some people use this property of vitamin C to help relieve their constipation, but in addition to vitamin C, this usually requires a high-fiber diet and adequate fluid intake.

In certain conditions, such as severe infections or inflammations, you may need extra ascorbate intravenously for adequate therapeutic effects. This route of administration avoids any potential loosening of the bowels. There are no other known side effects. There are no ascorbate-related problems with kidney stones or the destruction of vitamin B_{12}, as has been claimed by some vitamin antagonists. The claims that vitamin C has potential significant risks is not supported by scientific literature. Several flawed studies suggested possible theoretical side effects, but these were contradicted by other studies and have never been shown to relate to clinical effects.

A report in 1998 in the journal *Nature* showed that supposedly as little as 500 mg of vitamin C could increase the markers of oxidative damage to DNA. This study was severely criticized for its serious flaws. It was not placebo controlled, and the measurements were inadequate, outdated, and inaccurate. The conclusions were faulty for many reasons, partly because they did not report the balance of the pro- and antioxidative markers that they reported, and partly because they ignored the numerous other markers of oxidative protection and damage that they did not measure. This report was rejected for publication as a study and sort of sneaked in as a "brief report." It in no way diminishes the value of the hundreds of other studies that show vitamin C can reduce the risk of cancer. If I were isolated on a tropical island and could only have one vitamin supplement, I used to say it would be vitamin C, until I realized that on a tropical island I could probably get plenty of vitamin C in my diet. I realized that I would really like to take vitamin E, which is much harder to get from diet, as my first choice, or perhaps some coenzyme Q_{10} (and please, couldn't I just take a few others also?).

How to Take Vitamin C Vitamin C as ascorbic acid is available in tablet, capsule, or powder form. It is usually more convenient to take two or three tablets of 1,000 mg each, twice per day. If you prefer, the powder is easily dissolved in water or diluted juice; a quarter teaspoon usually equals approximately 1,000 mg. Ascorbic acid powder has a tart taste, and when added to diluted juice, makes the juice taste more like lemonade. Remember to rinse your mouth afterward, so the acid does not stay for long on the tooth enamel, where it might cause some erosion. For higher doses, the powder is easier to use (and cheaper). All these amounts are in addition to the 1,200 mg in the Basic Multiple, so if you are not taking that, you should try to get at least a total of 3,000 to 4,000 mg of vitamin C daily.

Buffered vitamin C is available if you do not like the sour taste of ascorbic acid. The buffered form has just over 1,000 mg per half teaspoon. The buffered vitamin C contains more minerals (usually calcium, magnesium, and potassium) and less vitamin C per teaspoon than plain vitamin C powder and is usually far more expensive.

Bioflavonoids are frequently added to some of the vitamin C tablets on the market. Although they do enhance the effectiveness of vitamin C, it is usually cheaper and more effective to take the flavonoids separately in order to have flexibility in adjusting the doses individually. (For more on the flavonoids, see chapter 8.)

A form of vitamin C called Ester-C has been heavily marketed for several years, claiming better absorption, staying longer in the cells or tissues, and better digestive tolerance. Dr. Pauling evaluated this product, and I spoke with him about it to ask his opinion. He said there was not good evidence that it provided extra benefits compared with other forms of vitamin C. He noted that it is quite a bit more expensive than the usual sources of ascorbate. In at least one research study, Ester-C has been shown to be inferior to plain ascorbic acid or ascorbate mixed with bioflavonoids. I am still not convinced of any extra benefit from Ester-C.

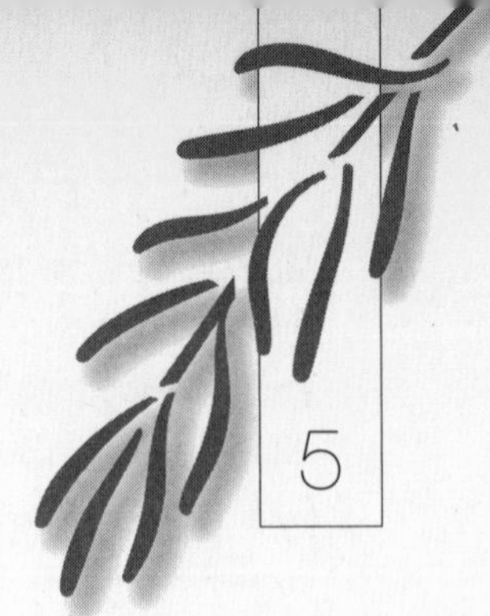

5

Mineral Supplements

MINERAL SUPPLEMENTS have a number of health benefits, although the valuable doses are more frequently closer to the RDA than those of other nutrients. Some of the minerals need to be more carefully balanced than the vitamins. There are both major minerals (or macro-minerals), which are those required in larger amounts, and trace minerals (or micro-minerals), which are required in very small daily amounts.

The major minerals are calcium, magnesium, sulfur, potassium, sodium, and phosphorus. The trace minerals include chromium, selenium, zinc, manganese, copper, iodine, and iron. You do not need to worry about getting too little sodium in the diet. Sodium chloride, or table salt, is far too abundant in the American diet, ranging from 5 to 13 g per day, when the need is for a mere 0.5 to 1 g per day. Potassium, on the other hand, is sometimes valuable as a supplement, especially if you do not eat a whole-foods diet.

There are also toxic minerals such as lead, mercury, aluminum, and cadmium that may interfere with the metabolism and absorption of the nutritional elements. The toxic minerals also have other harmful effects, and may increase the harmful effects of free radicals by interfering with the enzymes that detoxify them. There are only a few minerals that I recommend in amounts greater than the quantity in a good multivitamin/mineral combination such as the formula listed in chapter 2. (See page 24 for the Basic Multiple.)

Calcium

Calcium is probably the best-known mineral, due to all the publicity given to it by the dairy industry. In fact, you do not need dairy products at all to have adequate dietary calcium (after all, cows don't drink milk!). The need for calcium would probably be much lower than is publicized, if it weren't for the typical poor health habits in developed countries.

Too much sugar, caffeine, alcohol, meat, protein, and phosphate-containing sodas all contribute to the apparently higher need for calcium. They either decrease absorption of calcium or increase its excretion. Exercise improves calcium retention in the bones. Apparent requirements for calcium are much lower in many less-developed countries, where such inhibiting factors are less common. Absorption of calcium declines with age, and women absorb less than men do, regardless of age.

Calcium is the most abundant mineral in the body. Ninety-nine percent of the calcium in the body is found in the bones, where it gives strength to bone tissue. However, the free calcium is also important in many metabolic functions, including muscle contraction, nerve impulses, some hormone regulation, and blood clotting. Some studies show a lower incidence of bowel cancer and precancerous polyps in people who take calcium supplements, and it may help prevent osteoporosis when combined with a number of other equally important nutrients.

There is still controversy about the ideal dose of calcium. Whether women need more to prevent osteoporosis and what is the proper dose for cancer prevention are issues that have not been resolved. Calcium, but not dairy product sources, may lower heart disease risk.

How to Take Calcium Absorption of calcium is quite variable, depending on the previously listed factors and on stomach acidity. Many different forms of calcium are available. I believe the 500 mg of calcium (as ascorbate) present in Basic Multiple is adequate for most people who follow a healthy diet (not just minor variations of the typical American diet). Calcium supplements are better absorbed when taken with meals. If taken late in the day, it may help you sleep and reduce nighttime leg cramps (especially when balanced with magnesium).

When I recommend extra calcium, I usually suggest about 250 to 750 mg of calcium citrate, which is particularly well absorbed. Other forms of calcium, such as carbonate and lactate are sometimes well absorbed, but recent studies confirm that citrate is better. All are relatively inexpensive, but carbonate is least costly.

Chromium

Chromium is a trace mineral that is essential for the maintenance of normal blood sugar levels and the transport of sugar into the muscle cells for metabolism. It improves the function of insulin (the pancreatic hormone responsible for sugar regulation), which helps diabetics and hypoglycemics (people with fluctuating blood sugar levels, commonly called low blood sugar). Chromium has been shown to lower total cholesterol levels while at the same time raising the HDL (high-density lipoprotein), or good cholesterol.

Insulin regulation affects fat metabolism, and it has been claimed that chromium supplements can help weight loss, but there is not adequate evidence for this (the keys to any weight loss program remain diet and exercise). Diabetics need to take more than the usual supplementary amount of chromium for sugar regulation. This is not because they have a deficiency in their diets, but because they are resistant to the effects of chromium.

Chromium is a part of the glucose tolerance factor (GTF), a biologically active substance manufactured in the body, which regulates sugar metabolism. GTF is thought to be a combination of chromium with niacin and several amino acids, but the structure of GTF itself has not been clearly characterized. However, it appears that the material that your body produces is more active than any of the manufactured substances called GTF.

How to Take Chromium I usually recommend the 200 mcg in Basic Multiple, and this is generally enough for most people. Additional chromium supplements are available as GTF-chromium (which is not actual glucose tolerance factor), chromium niacinate, and chromium picolinate, all of which are effective. People have heavily debated the value of the picolinate compared to the GTF or the niacinate forms, usually because they have a financial interest in one or the other. It appears that all supplemental forms of chromium are clinically active, with minor metabolic differences.

If there are problems with diabetes, high cholesterol, or weight control, I will commonly recommend an additional 400 to 800 mcg per day. I use the GTF-chromium or a combination of GTF with chromium picolinate, available in 200- to 300-mcg capsules. Chromium is also available in 1,000-mcg tablets, which is useful for people who prefer taking fewer tablets and need the high doses for diabetes control.

Iron

There is more iron in the body than any other trace element. It is mostly present in the red blood cells as a part of hemoglobin, the molecule that carries oxygen. Iron is also necessary for the activity of a number of enzymes. A deficiency of iron causes anemia, resulting in fatigue and listlessness. Perhaps because of the other functions of iron, low levels may cause fatigue without obvious anemia.

Too much iron can stimulate the production of free radicals, so it is important to be cautious with both iron supplements and food sources. Studies in Finland and elsewhere have shown that excess iron accumulation is a strong risk factor for the development of heart disease. It is also associated with increased cancer rates. Much of this excess iron comes from meat in the diet.

I only recommend supplements of iron if there is a demonstrated need for it, based on clinical and laboratory evidence. Because of poor diet, iron deficiency is quite common. There are increased needs for iron during pregnancy, and infants may also need extra iron. Iron is responsible for many poisonings when children find bottles of iron supplements meant for adults. Make sure the bottles have childproof caps (although these are sometimes the kind that only kids can open), and be sure to keep the bottles out of the reach of children.

How to Take Iron Iron supplements are available in many forms. The most common form, iron sulfate, causes constipation and digestive upset and is not the best absorbed. I usually recommend iron carbonyl—the safest form of iron—in a timed-release, 50-mg tablet. The dose needs to be individualized, and a typical dose is one to three tablets per day until the deficiency is cured. Iron is best absorbed when taken with vitamin C supplements or foods that are rich in vitamin C, such as oranges.

Magnesium

Magnesium is a major mineral that is frequently ignored in medical circles, but it is extremely important. Recently, the medical community has taken a much greater interest in the therapeutic role of magnesium, especially in heart disease. It helps normal heart and muscle function, neurologic function, and normal metabolism of fats, and it reduces arrhythmias of the heart, high blood pressure, anxiety, insomnia, and pre-eclampsia (toxemia of pregnancy). It is also an important component of bone, and it is involved in over three hundred enzyme systems.

Magnesium is an important part of the treatment of premenstrual syndrome and menstrual cramps. It is commonly low in the diet and in body tissues. I was surprised when I first learned about nutrition—after medical school—to reread this fact about magnesium in my medical school biochemistry text. It was never taught to me in school. The official requirements for magnesium are 280 mg and 350 mg per day for women and men, respectively. I believe that a healthier recommendation is closer to 500 to 1,000 mg per day, especially for people with heart or neurological problems.

Diuretic drugs cause loss of magnesium in the urine (in addition to the better-publicized loss of potassium). Magnesium is also wasted by consumption of caffeine, alcohol, and sugar. Low levels are related to fatigue (including chronic fatigue syndrome), allergies, nervousness and irritability, and hyperactivity and bedwetting in children. It is available in a variety of compounds, and they vary in absorption.

When patients are first starting therapy for muscle spasms, acute pain, acute asthma attacks, or anxiety, I often treat them with intravenous magnesium supplements (combined with vitamin C and B complex). It is safer, cheaper, and more effective than many of the drugs used for these same purposes. This treatment is not well known among physicians, perhaps because it is too inexpensive to be publicized by drug companies.

How to Take Magnesium I usually recommend taking 500 to 1,000 mg of magnesium each day. The Basic Multiple contains 500 mg of magnesium, and in addition I might recommend 100 to 200 mg twice per day as magnesium aspartate, which is well absorbed. For heart patients or asthma patients, I will sometimes recommend even up to 1,500 mg. High doses may cause some loosening of the bowels, but magnesium has no other side effects unless abused in extremely high doses (such as by taking antacids in large amounts).

Patients with serious kidney disorders who can't eliminate magnesium properly must be very cautious about their intake of extra magnesium, which can accumulate in the blood.

Dolomite is one source of both calcium and magnesium. If your digestion is good, it may be well absorbed. In the past some dolomite supplements were contaminated with heavy metals such as lead, but this is not a recent problem. The ratio of calcium to magnesium (2:1) was thought to be ideal at one time, but many of my colleagues now believe that an equal amount (or even more magnesium) is a better balance. This is still not a completely resolved issue.

Selenium

Selenium is a required trace mineral that is important in the fight against excess exposure to free radicals. Adequate intake is associated with a decreased risk of cancer, including colon and breast cancer, and it reduces the incidence of heart disease. Selenium also helps to displace mercury, a toxic heavy metal, from the tissues. Tuna and swordfish, which may have high levels of mercury, also usually have high levels of selenium to balance it. Low levels of selenium may lead to seborrheic dermatitis and dandruff. Selenium is another of the nutrients helpful with macular degeneration.

Many people have a low intake of selenium, especially in those geographical areas where the soil selenium has been depleted as a result of ice-age glacial activity. Many areas of the world have low soil selenium, including regions of China, Eastern Europe, the Middle East, Scandinavia, New Zealand, and many areas of the United States, including the Northeast (whereas in the Midwest the soil selenium level is quite variable). In these areas, the incidence of cancers is higher. Critics of selenium supplementation have said that even though we live in areas with low soil selenium, the food supply comes from all over the country and the world, so local conditions should not make any difference. They have not adequately answered the epidemiological data, which shows that the local amount of selenium in the soil does make a difference in the disease rate, and that supplements might well make a difference in cancer incidence.

Selenium is a component of an important antioxidant enzyme—glutathione peroxidase. This is essential for the full activity of vitamin E, because it helps to regenerate the unoxidized form of the vitamin. This is another example of how antioxidants work together to provide free-radical protection. Deficiency of selenium may also lead to low thyroid function because it is necessary for an enzyme that converts one form of the hormone (thyroxine or T4) to the active form (T3). Severe deficiency can lead to an inflammation of the heart muscle.

How to Take Selenium The Basic Multiple formula contains 200 mcg of selenium, the basic amount I suggest. I often recommend an additional 200 to 400 mcg per day for patients at high risk of cancer or heart disease, or for those people who want a more vigorous free-radical protective program. It is available in 200-mcg tablets. Any of the available forms of supplemental selenium is effective.

Zinc

Zinc is a trace mineral necessary for normal growth and development, and sexual maturation. It is also a cofactor for the activity of many enzymes. A large concentration of zinc is found in the skin, nails, retina, and testes. It is also a component of a special antioxidant enzyme called *superoxide dismutase* (SOD) that is manufactured in the body. (Different forms of this enzyme are also dependent on copper and manganese.) SOD is an important oxygen-free-radical scavenger. (For a full discussion of free radicals, see chapter 1.) Zinc and copper need to be taken in balance, since they compete with each other for absorption. There are different opinions on just what a healthy balance is, but a ratio of about 10:1 (zinc to copper) is reasonable.

Supplements of zinc help with burn and wound healing, enhancement of immune function, and the treatment of acne and other skin disorders. It is one of several nutrients helpful in macular degeneration (loss of vision in the most sensitive area of the retina). Zinc lozenges dissolved in the mouth help to cut short viral infections of the upper respiratory tract, including the common cold. Apparently the direct contact helps to kill viruses.

Zinc is a very important nutrient for mental health and is sometimes useful in the treatment of schizophrenia, and autism. (For these patients I also suggest supplements of magnesium, niacin, pyridoxine, and essential fatty acids). It has recently been reported in the *Journal of the American Medical Association* that supplementing the diet with zinc during pregnancy (25 mg per day) has resulted in larger, healthier babies. This amount is commonly present in prenatal vitamins and other supplements.

Zinc has been used therapeutically in very high doses (up to 150 mg per day) to treat prostate enlargement, but such doses may not be necessary if you combine this treatment with essential fatty acids, botanical extracts, and other nutrients. With high doses of zinc, special attention has to be paid to the proper mineral balance in the body, especially copper. The higher doses may decrease the level of good cholesterol (HDL). Zinc may be helpful in the removal of lead and cadmium, which it can displace from tissues.

How to Take Zinc The usual doses that I recommend are in the form of zinc gluconate, which is well absorbed. Basic Multiple contains 30 mg of zinc (along with 3 mg of copper for proper balance). I may use an additional 50 to 100 mg of zinc per day for specific conditions. Patients receiving chelation therapy (an intravenous therapy for vascular disease and heavy metal excess) usually need extra zinc—typically 50 mg daily—because so much is excreted in the urine as a result of the treatment.

Zinc gluconate supplements are commonly available in 15- to 50-mg tablets. The typical dose in the lozenges for colds is about 15 mg. Taking several lozenges per day can reduce the duration of the symptoms. Although there are data showing some enhanced absorption from zinc picolinate, the actual clinical effects are apparently just as good with the less expensive forms, such as zinc gluconate. Chelated zinc is another available supplement. It is usually more expensive without having a clear advantage over other forms.

Other Trace Elements

The other trace minerals—copper, manganese, molybdenum, boron, vanadium, cobalt, and iodine—are also important for health, even though only extremely small amounts are required.

Boron, in a dose of 3 mg per day, has been shown to help retain bone density in menopausal women, perhaps because it can increase serum levels of estrogen. Since this information was published, the daily 3-mg dose of boron is now found more often in multivitamin preparations.

Cobalt is known primarily for its functions related to its presence in vitamin B_{12}, although there is a relationship of non-B_{12} cobalt to certain enzyme functions. Cobalt appears to be related to red blood cell formation independent of its being a part of vitamin B_{12}. Older studies suggest that large amounts can lower blood pressure in hypertensive patients, but no recent research has been done to either dispute or support this effect. Some research suggests that it is important for thyroid function. I am not familiar with any available supplements of cobalt other than that in B_{12}.

Copper is another mineral essential for SOD activity, as well as connective tissue maintenance and immune function. Low copper levels can lead to high blood cholesterol. Excess copper has been considered a problem with mental illness, elevated blood pressure, and irritability, but many clinicians now feel that low copper levels are a more common problem than excess copper.

Iodine is the critical element in thyroid gland hormone, and it also has some special therapeutic uses. It is used medically to treat goiter (swelling of the thyroid with low thyroid function) if the goiter is the result of low iodine intake, which is very rare in this country. It is advisable that a knowledgeable health practitioner recommend iodine supplements.

Manganese is essential for bone and cartilage formation and for the function of one form of the antioxidant enzyme SOD (superoxide dismutase), which protects the mitochondrial membranes (those little intracellular engines again) from oxidation. It is also a cofactor for a number of other enzymes, and it is yet another nutrient helpful with macular degeneration. A common dose range is from 6 to 20 mg daily.

Vanadium may be an essential mineral, but little is known about its nutritional importance. Supplemental vanadium, as vanadyl sulfate in doses that go beyond nutritional levels, is valuable for diabetics. It acts like insulin in these amounts, ranging up to 100 mg daily. It also lowers cholesterol at these doses. Vanadium also appears to improve bone density by stimulating bone-forming cells. There is little long-term research on vanadium, but I have seen diabetic patients taking 50 to 150 mg daily show improvement in their blood sugar control.

The amounts of these trace minerals in the Basic Multiple are generally sufficient for most health programs. Sometimes people do need extra copper or manganese, and diabetics may benefit from supplemental vanadyl sulfate. If your multi does not have one of these, they are available as separate supplements.

There are some other essential trace elements about which less is known, such as silicon, tin, germanium, and nickel, and they are not generally included in supplements.

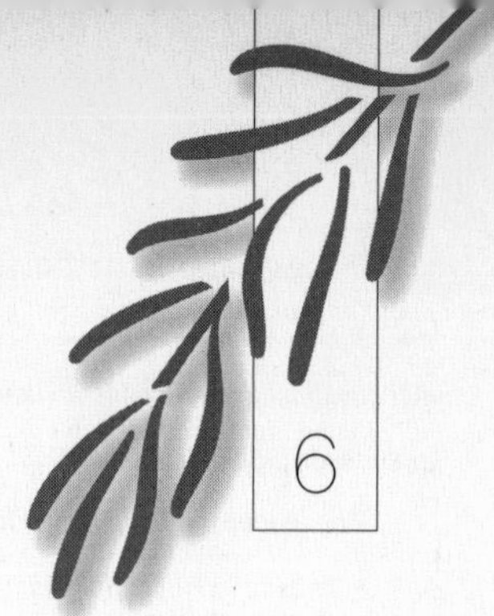

Dietary Fats and Essential Fatty Acids

ONLY RECENTLY HAVE WE DEVELOPED an understanding of the role of dietary fats in health. Fats are a source of energy (or calories—too many in most cases) and provide structural protection around organs. As we'll see, they are also important components of cell membranes and precursors of important regulatory molecules.

Types of Fats

Fats are made up of long chains of carbon atoms with attached hydrogen atoms, and some oxygen atoms at the end. Each carbon has four link sites to attach to the neighboring carbon, a hydrogen atom, or other atoms. Some neighboring carbon atoms are double-linked to each other (a "double bond"), taking up two of the bonds where there could have been two more hydrogen atoms. These fats are called *unsaturated* because they don't have all the hydrogen atoms they could have. Fats with one double bond are called *monounsaturated* fats. Fats with more than one double bond are called *polyunsaturated* fats.

Fats can come from animal or vegetable sources. Oils are simply fats that are liquid at room temperature because they are unsaturated. Saturated fats are solid at room temperature, and monounsaturated fats (abundant in olive oil) are liquid but become solid if you put them in the refrigerator. Some saturated fats have been artificially saturated, or *hydrogenated.* This refers to the addition of hydrogen atoms to some of the double-bonded carbon atoms through reactions facilitated by heat and catalysts. They are usually called "partially hydrogenated" oils because they are not completely saturated with hydrogen. This is how they make margarine and shortening.

Both those fats that occur naturally as saturated fats (animal fats, coconut and palm oils) and those that are artificially hydrogenated are solid at room temperature. The artificially saturated fats contain damaging substances called *trans* fats, which do not occur naturally. (More about them later.) Animal fat and partially hydrogenated oils can increase inflammatory reactions and elevate the amount of cholesterol and fat in the blood. Vegetarian diets generally contain very little saturated fat, aside from possibly coconut oil and palm oil, and some vegetarians do eat dairy products or eggs. (*Vegans* are strict vegetarians who eat no animal products.)

Trans Fatty Acids

Let's get back to *trans* fatty acids. In their natural state, edible oils exist in a specific three-dimensional spatial configuration referred to as *cis.* When oils are highly processed during hydrogenation with heat and catalysts, they are partially converted to a different configuration called *trans.* These trans fatty acids do not participate in the normal pathways of fatty acid metabolism. They may actually block the conversion of the natural cis fats to their active metabolites. Partially saturated or partly hydrogenated oil almost invariably contains trans fats. Oils that have been made into margarine contain significant amounts of trans fats, although food processors have made recent efforts to reduce the trans fat content of some margarine brands. Most processed foods and baked goods contain partially hydrogenated oils (or shortening), and there is now a significant amount of these abnormal fats in the Western diet. Trans fats increase the risk of developing heart disease and possibly cancer more than natural saturated fats. In addition, trans fats may interfere with normal immune function through effects on prostaglandin production. I would suggest that you avoid trans fats in your diet; they generally only occur in processed foods that are not very good for you anyway.

Essential Fatty Acids

Some polyunsaturated fats are required in the diet and are therefore called *essential fatty acids,* or EFAs. These fats are essential for many reasons. They are an important component of cell membranes. These membranes allow passage of molecules in and out of cells and maintain receptors for hormones. Fats are also the building blocks for hormones. EFAs may be converted into derivatives called *prostaglandins,* important hormonelike regulatory substances.

Good health is dependent on a proper balance of the different types of fats. Watch out for the spelling of the two essential fatty acids: linol*ei*c and linol*en*ic. *Linoleic* acid is an *omega-6* unsaturated fat, with its first double bond at the sixth position along the carbon chain. It is found in corn and beans. Linoleic acid is converted through a series of steps to a regulatory substance called prostaglandin E_1. Prostaglandins regulate many metabolic functions. Minute amounts can cause significant changes in blood pressure, blood clotting, cholesterol levels, inflammatory responses, allergies, hormone activity, immune function, neurologic function, and more. Prostaglandin E_1 decreases the tendency of platelets to clump together, decreases inflammation, stabilizes blood sugar, and decreases cholesterol. It decreases spasms in arterial and other involuntary muscle.

A deficiency of omega-6 EFA may result in eczema, premenstrual syndrome, breast pain and lumpiness, inflammation, and autoimmune problems, hyperactivity in children, and hypertension. Many people have adequate intake of these oils but inefficient conversion to the active prostaglandins. Specifically, individuals with a history of allergy, high cholesterol, diabetes, high alcohol intake, trans fat intake, chemical exposures, or specific nutrient deficiencies (particularly of magnesium and vitamin B_6) may have difficulty with conversion. In these cases the metabolic block can be bypassed by taking supplements of GLA (*gamma-linol*en*ic* acid—that's right, linol*ei*c is converted to gamma-linol*en*ic, just to confuse you), which helps treat the problems listed above.

The other EFA is *alpha-linolenic* acid, which is an *omega-3* oil. This oil is even more unsaturated (has more double bonds), with the first double bond at the third position in the carbon chain. This molecular structure gives the oil different properties. Omega-3 oils predominate in fish oils, flaxseeds (linseeds), and some nuts, particularly walnuts. Omega-3 oils play a significant role in reducing the risk of coronary heart disease. Scientists have confirmed that populations that regularly consume more fish have a lower incidence of heart disease. These oils decrease the tendency of platelets to clump together, a reaction involved in the development of atherosclerosis as well as the precipitation of heart attacks. Omega-3 oils also decrease triglycerides, cholesterol, and inflammatory reactions.

There is evidence that a deficiency of omega-3 oils is associated with various skin disorders, arthritis and joint stiffness, prostate problems, irritable bowel syndrome, premenstrual syndrome, depression, phobias, and schizophrenia. These oils have a short shelf life, and they are generally removed from our food supply through processing for manufacturers' convenience. Deficiencies are therefore common.

It is important to have the right amount of EFAs in the diet or as supplements. If you do use nutritious oils as part of the diet, don't go overboard. They are high in calories, and you don't need much for good nutrition. All other animals get their EFAs from foods, such as seeds, nuts, and grains, but you may need therapeutic levels. However, you don't want to gain weight from too many calories.

The metabolism and clinical use of the essential fatty acids has been one of the remarkable developments in medicine in the past two decades. The education of physicians regarding these oils is due in part to the work of two physicians, David Horrobin, M.D., and Donald Rudin, M.D., who have done research, scoured the literature, and reported on the physiology of fats and oils. Many open-minded clinicians who have tried supplements of these essential fatty acids as treatments for their patients have been impressed with the results. Essential fatty acids are now an important component of nutritional therapeutics. They are beneficial for a variety of clinical problems. They are safe, easy to take, and relatively inexpensive.

Essential Fatty Acid Supplements: EPA and DHA

EPA stands for eicosapentaenoic acid, so it is obvious why we call it simply EPA. This is a fish oil concentrate of omega-3 oil that has already started its conversion to prostaglandin E_3. Fish oil supplements also contain DHA (docosahexaenoic acid), another omega-3 essential fatty acid, which has similar properties.

Fish oil supplements have been shown to reduce inflammation, especially in arthritis, and to reduce rejection reactions after organ transplants, without the side effects of some of the antirejection drugs. They also lower cholesterol levels and reduce platelet stickiness. This reduces the risk of clots inside the blood vessels. They can help with some of the symptoms of premenstrual syndrome, bowel dysfunction, and mental illness. Fish oil supplements can lower cholesterol levels in the blood, help to lower blood pressure, and reduce excessive blood clotting (platelet activity). It is helpful in heart and blood vessel disease. DHA is specifically important for the neurological development of infants, who may need supplements if they are not fed breast milk, which is rich in DHA.

How to Take Essential Fatty Acid Supplements The usual therapeutic dose of fish oils ranges from 3 to 12 g per day. Capsules of 1,000 mg (containing 180 mg of EPA and 120 mg of DHA) are commonly available, and there are also some supplements with a higher concentration of these active oils. Sometimes higher doses are used in studies, for example, on arthritis, but with comprehensive diet and supplement programs it is usually possible to achieve beneficial effects with lower doses. I usually recommend starting on two to four of the 1,000-mg capsules per day, and may increase the dose if the response is not adequate.

Flaxseed Oil

Flaxseeds are another good source of omega-3 oil. Many of their effects are similar to those of fish oil, but because they have not yet gone through the first step in conversion they may not be as helpful in some situations. Supplements of flaxseed oil are useful in a variety of skin disorders, including psoriasis, and digestive problems, including spastic colon and probably inflammatory bowel disease. Some claims have been made for benefits in other inflammatory diseases, as well as cancer and immune system problems.

How to Take Flaxseed Oil Usual doses of flaxseed oil are 1 to 3 tablespoons per day for therapeutic purposes, reducing this to 1 to 3 teaspoons after the desired effect is achieved. It is available in 8.8- and 17.6-ounce bottles. Some manufacturers process the oil in an inert gas environment, and then package it in opaque bottles without oxygen because it is very easily oxidized if exposed to heat and light. I recommend keeping it in the freezer until it is opened, and then in the refrigerator. (After having been in the freezer, it will take a few minutes to liquefy.) It is a good idea never to cook with flaxseed oil because of its sensitivity to heat, but you may safely add it to hot foods after cooking.

Flaxseeds themselves are a good source of the omega-3 oil and a large amount of fiber, especially soluble fiber and lignans. Each tablespoon of seeds contains about one teaspoon of oil. The fiber in flaxseeds is an effective treatment for both constipation and diarrhea, and it helps to eliminate toxins. Grinding the seeds only for immediate use (in a small electric coffee mill or seed grinder) provides the freshest source of the oil. I like to grind up some flaxseeds and add them to a blender drink with frozen banana, other fruit, diluted juice, and a few other ingredients, such as brewer's yeast, powdered green food mixtures, and glutamine powder.

Gamma-Linolenic Acid (GLA)

Gamma-linolenic acid, or GLA, is found in evening primrose oil, borage oil, and black currant oil. GLA is produced by enzyme action on the linoleic acid that is essential in the diet. It is the result of the first step in conversion to the beneficial prostaglandin PGE_1, bypassing the metabolic blockages mentioned above. Supplements have anti-inflammatory effects because they lead to increased production of PGE_1.

Many studies have shown remarkable benefits from supplements of

GLA. It helps relieve premenstrual symptoms, eczema, asthma, and autoimmune disorders. It can lower blood pressure in hypertensives by relaxing blood vessel muscles, and it decreases excessive blood clotting. It helps to regulate hormonal function through its effect on production and release of hormones, and through control of hormone activity at the target organs. GLA has been shown to help in alcoholism, diabetes, acne, hyperactivity, and numerous other conditions. Although it sounds miraculous, its effects are easily explainable based on well-known nutritional biochemistry.

How to Take GLA I usually recommend the borage oil source of GLA, since it is the most cost-effective and concentrated, meaning that fewer pills are necessary. It comes in 1,200-mg capsules, which contain 240 mg of GLA. One per day is usually adequate. Evening primrose oil is the best-studied source of GLA, but not the most cost-effective. It contains 40 mg of GLA per 500-mg capsule (usual dose—six per day). Black currant oil contains about 80 mg per capsule, and three per day is an adequate dose. After therapeutic results, the dose may be lowered for maintenance.

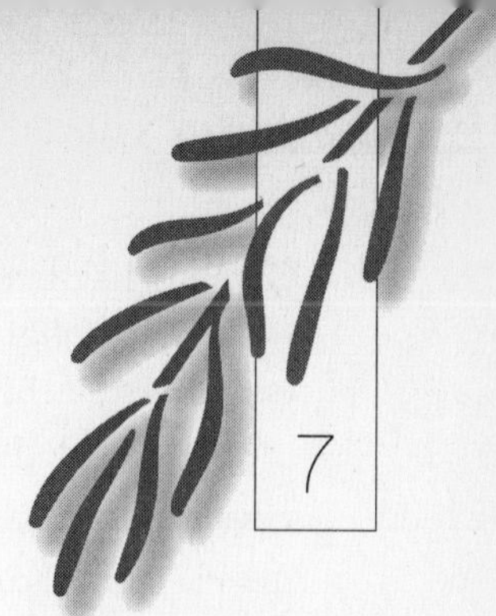

7

Amino Acids

AMINO ACIDS ARE THE BUILDING BLOCKS of protein molecules. They get their name from a nitrogen-hydrogen combination called an amine, or amino group attached to the molecule. There are eight essential amino acids—the kind you must get in the diet because your body cannot manufacture them. Most people get enough of the amino acids that they need from the protein that they eat. In fact, most Americans get too much protein, especially animal protein, so they have an abundance of amino acids for building body proteins. Most of the amino acids from foods go into the manufacture of the different proteins of the body, or they are burned for energy, and any excess is converted to fat.

Some amino acids are also used for other purposes, such as providing the base molecule for the manufacture of hormones or nerve transmitters that carry the nerve signal from one nerve in a chain to the next one. Serotonin is a nerve transmitter derived from the amino acid tryptophan, and thyroid hormone is derived from another amino acid—tyrosine. The hormone insulin is made up of a chain of amino acids.

Amino acids are also nitrogen sources for the nucleic acids (DNA and RNA) of our genes. Enzymes are made up of protein molecules. Several of the amino acids are therapeutically useful. Some amino acids are essential (required in the diet). Some of them are produced in the body but in less-than-ideal amounts. In these situations, supplements are extremely valuable. Also, in certain health problems the need for therapeutic levels of specific amino acids rises dramatically for production of the hormones or neurotransmitters, or for other specific healing benefits. These specific amounts are usually not supplied sufficiently by the protein in the diet.

Because amino acids are present in large amounts in food, it is common for supplements to be more effective when taken separately from meals containing other protein sources. Since they are not given for their protein value as much as for their precursor value, they may be "drowned out" by other amino acids from typical high-protein foods and be pushed into protein formation. Unfortunately, people frequently forget to take supplements separately from mealtimes, so you are more likely to take amino acid supplements successfully if you do so with your meals. Taking at least some of the dose at bedtime and on arising is a reasonable alternative and may be easier to remember. Dietary supplements that you do not remember to take are 100 percent ineffective.

Amino Acids and Proteins

In the United States and other developed countries, many people actually consume too much protein, although not necessarily in the right balance. Too much protein creates a nitrogen overload on the liver and kidneys, and people with liver or kidney disorders must be extremely cautious about consuming any extra amino acids. If you take therapeutic levels of amino acids, it is usually a good idea to reduce other protein sources (unless you are already on a relatively low-protein vegetarian diet).

Amino acid names are usually preceded by the letter *L*, which refers to their ability to rotate the plane of polarized light in a "left-handed" direction. This is the usual natural form of the molecule. (The *D* form is normally only used as a supplement in the DL-form of phenylalanine.)

L-Arginine

L-arginine is a nonessential amino acid (or semi-essential or "conditionally essential"—needed in some conditions) that is a precursor of nitric oxide. Nitric oxide is an arterial wall muscle relaxant (also known as endothelial-derived relaxing factor) that helps to open up the arteries. As a consequence, arginine supplements may help with hypertension and coronary artery disease. As an example of the importance of nitric oxide, the drug nitroglycerin is useful for the treatment of angina pectoris (chest pain from coronary artery disease) because it releases nitric oxide.

Arginine has also been shown to reduce chemical carcinogenesis (production of cancer). It has been touted as a muscle builder because of its potential to stimulate the release of growth hormone from the pituitary gland. Some reports suggest that the balance of arginine and lysine (another amino acid) is important in recurrence rates of infections with Herpes simplex virus. Too much arginine may precipitate outbreaks of herpes, and thus it must sometimes be balanced with supplements of lysine.

Arginine can enhance hormone release (prolactin, insulin, and glucagon), improve immunity, and increase the rate of wound healing after trauma, burns, or surgery. Studies have shown that patients who take arginine supplements need to stay less time in the hospital after surgery. It may be of help in asthma, too, because the nitric oxide it produces is also a relaxant of the bronchial (airway) muscles. Some research suggests that arginine can enhance erections in men with sexual dysfunction because the nitric oxide released by arginine is essential to the erectile process. Some have even referred to arginine as "natural Viagra."

How to Take Arginine I have used 500 to 1,000 mg of arginine twice per day, but higher doses may help some conditions. Much of the research shows benefits for hypertension, heart disease, and immune function with doses of 2,000 to 6,000 mg per day. Similar doses are useful for erectile dysfunction. With combined supplements and diet, the lower dose may be adequate. Arginine is commonly available in 500-mg capsules and is also available as a powder to make it easier to take higher doses.

L-Carnitine

L-carnitine is sometimes called vitamin B_t, but it is not a true vitamin as you manufacture it in the body. It is an amino acid derivative necessary for the metabolism of fat in the cells. Fat is burned for energy in cells by the mitochondria. A membrane surrounds the mitochondria, and carnitine is essential for the passage of fat across this membrane. As a consequence, L-carnitine enhances the burning of fat, lowers the triglyceride (fat) level in the blood, and may make it easier for some people to lose weight.

Your body makes carnitine from the amino acids lysine and methionine (requiring vitamins C, B_6, B_3, and iron), so it is not considered essential, but the production is often low, especially in disease states. L-carnitine levels are high in muscle, especially heart muscle, but it is very low in the muscle of patients with arteriosclerosis (hardening of the arteries). Supplementation with L-carnitine increases its tissue levels and improves the skeletal and heart muscle energy.

Larger doses of L-carnitine (1,000–2,000 mg per day) are effective for the relief of angina pectoris (heart pain due to diminished oxygen). L-carnitine is especially valuable if given for a period of time before symptoms occur. In allowing more burning of fat, it reduces the muscle dependency on glucose. When glucose is burned with too little oxygen (as in hardening of the arteries or intense muscle activity), the extra lactic acid produced leads to increased pain (as in a racer's calf muscles). For the same reason, it can improve energy, stamina, and recovery rate in athletes.

L-carnitine is also useful for patients with hardening of the arteries to the legs, which leads to pain on walking called "intermittent claudication." Walking distance before pain starts is much longer when patients take carnitine supplements, usually in the range of 2000 mg daily.

How to Take L-Carnitine I usually recommend capsules of 250 to 500 mg, and suggest taking 1,000 to 2,000 mg per day for patients with heart disease. Much higher levels have been given experimentally with no side effects, and they appear to be particularly helpful in heart patients and those with intermittent claudication. Carnitine is quite safe. Athletic performance is improved even in trained endurance athletes with doses of 2,000 mg daily.

L-Glutamine

L-glutamine is the most abundant free amino acid in the bloodstream. It helps build muscle, especially in times of stress or illness. It is a major transporter of nitrogen, an important energy source for the intestinal lining cells, and it is essential for immune function. Glutamine is critically important in the healing of peptic ulcers and inflammatory bowel disease, and in treating diarrhea. Supplements of glutamine may dramatically improve recovery after surgery or trauma, and it can hasten the healing of wounds.

L-glutamine reduces cravings that result from low blood sugar and also helps to improve memory. The brain usually burns sugar (glucose) as its main fuel. When sugar levels are low, neurologic and psychiatric symptoms can develop. However, the brain can use glutamine as an alternative fuel to decrease those mental symptoms. It can reduce depression and fatigue. Glutamine is also an important antioxidant precursor, since the body uses it to make glutathione, an antioxidant enzyme.

How to Take L-Glutamine L-glutamine supplements are readily available in 500-mg capsules, and it is also available as a pure powder that can be mixed with water or diluted juice when very high doses are needed. (When looking for supplements, be sure to specify L-glutamine, not glutamate or glutamic acid.) I will frequently recommend two or three capsules twice per day (2,000 to 3,000 mg total), and sometimes up to 4,500 mg per day. Higher doses of glutamine are useful for more severe inflammatory bowel conditions, wasting diseases, and ulcers. Researchers are still evaluating the use of high doses of glutamine for immune function disorders such as AIDS, and the preliminary results are very promising.

L-Lysine

L-lysine is an essential amino acid. It is therapeutic for the treatment of herpes viruses, especially when properly balanced with a relatively low arginine intake. If you take arginine supplements and are susceptible to herpes (cold sores or fever blisters), you should probably take some lysine at the same time. It has been suggested that high doses of L-lysine may stimulate increased production of cholesterol by the liver, but in my experience this is not very common. On the other hand, lysine is a precursor of L-carnitine, and L-carnitine helps to lower triglyceride and cholesterol levels. There is some evidence that L-lysine supplements can help with the treatment of heart and blood vessel disease (atherosclerosis).

How to Take L-Lysine The usual dose of L-lysine for prevention of herpes is 500 to 1,000 mg per day. When an outbreak occurs, the dose may be increased to 2,000 to 4,000 mg per day. With this dose, the lesions heal faster and the recurrences are less frequent. For heart disease, the recommendation is 1,500 mg daily. It comes in 500-mg capsules.

L-Taurine

L-taurine is one of the few sulfur-containing amino acids (others are cysteine and methionine). It is unlike other amino acids in that it is not incorporated into proteins. Although it is not essential, because it can be made from cysteine, it is not always made in adequate amounts for optimal physiological function. Sulfur carriers are important antioxidants. L-taurine is important for solubility of the bile and may help prevent or treat gallstones. It is also involved in stabilizing cell membranes, and it therefore affects nerve conduction and hypersensitivity.

Taurine has a role in balancing sodium and potassium in the heart muscle and other cells, and it helps increase the strength of the heartbeat in congestive heart failure. In some fad liquid-protein diets of the late 1970s and early 1980s, serious complications resulted because they contained inadequate taurine. This prevented proper uptake of potassium into the heart muscle, leading to arrhythmias. Clinical experience shows that taurine is helpful for patients with various heart rhythm problems (skipped beats or palpitations). It also helps to lower blood pressure if it is abnormally high.

Taurine levels are high in the retina of the eye, where it is concentrated in the cells that receive light, and it is likely to be helpful in treating and preventing age-related macular degeneration. It also helps prevent damage from ultraviolet light and some toxic substances.

How to Take L-Taurine Taurine is available as 500-mg capsules, and I usually recommend one or two of these twice per day for heart-failure or arrhythmia patients. The same amount has been helpful for some seizure disorders. For preventing eye disorders, one or two capsules may be adequate (although sometimes it is given intravenously as treatment for more serious macular degeneration).

In reviewing the research, you will find that up to twelve capsules per day have been used in heart disease studies. However, these doses may not be needed when taurine is used in combination with other nutrients. This is a common finding in clinical practice, in which synergistic effects allow for lower doses of individual supplements, as compared with medical studies in which a single substance is used to provide clearer research results.

L-Tryptophan and 5-HTP

L-tryptophan is an essential amino acid that is an important precursor to both serotonin and melatonin. As a precursor of serotonin, a neurotransmitter, it has profound effects on brain function. Increasing brain levels of serotonin with supplements of tryptophan has relieved both depression and insomnia, and it has also been shown to help with bulimia.

Some of the most popular recent drug prescriptions for depression (Prozac, Zoloft) are effective specifically because they result in increased levels of serotonin in the brain, but tryptophan produces the same results without the risk of the side effects seen with those medications. Some people have speculated that the reason the FDA removed tryptophan from the market in 1989 had more to do with its competition with drugs than with the isolated, temporary contamination problem in one batch of the product. (See inset on page 75, "FDA Bans Trytophan.")

Although tryptophan is not currently available as an over-the-counter supplement for human consumption as of this writing, the common dosage form that was available before the FDA ban was as capsules of 500 mg. I have recommended doses of 1,000 to 4,000 mg per day, usually starting with 1,000 mg twice per day, including one dose at bedtime. Unfortunately, many patients who depended on tryptophan to keep them in good mental health, or for restorative sleep, have been forced either to suffer or to take medications since it is no longer available as a dietary supplement. Let me emphasize that these drugs frequently have side effects not seen with tryptophan. It is my honest hope that tryptophan will soon be back on the market. It is currently available as a prescription from compounding pharmacies if you can find a doctor willing to prescribe it.

5-Hydroxy-L-Tryptophan

5-hydroxy-L-tryptophan is a tryptophan derivative (5-HTP) that may be even better than tryptophan as a dietary supplement, and it is readily available without a prescription from your health food supplier. It has the same effects in that it is also a precursor for the production of serotonin. Because it is one metabolic step closer to serotonin, the effective dose is lower than with L-tryptophan.

5-HTP is effective in the treatment of depression and insomnia. It has also been successful in treating migraine headaches and fibromyalgia syndrome, which is similar to chronic fatigue, with symptoms of fatigue, muscle and joint aches and pains, tenderness, malaise, low resistance to infection.

How to take 5-HTP The typical dose of 5-HTP is 50 mg twice a day, for the treatment of insomnia, depression, and anxiety. For migraines and fibromyalgia syndrome, the doses range from 100 to 400 mg per day. Sometimes the higher doses are used for depression. I usually recommend taking at least one of the doses at bedtime, especially if insomnia is a problem.

Phenylalanine

Phenylalanine is an essential amino acid that, in addition to its role in protein formation, is a precursor of several important metabolites. It can be made into another amino acid called tyrosine, and from there into the adrenal hormones, including norepinephrine. Norepinephrine (structurally similar to adrenaline) is a neurotransmitter.

Tyrosine is also metabolized into melanin, the skin pigment. Metabolic addition of iodine to tyrosine leads to the formation of thyroid hormone.

FDA Bans Tryptophan

In 1989 the United States Food and Drug Administration (FDA) removed a very valuable amino acid—tryptophan—from the supplement market because of a single contaminated batch that was imported from a single manufacturer in Japan. The contaminant was soon revealed to be the result of a new manufacturing process, and the problem was solved. This information was published in the *American Journal of Epidemiology* and the *Journal of the American Medical Association* as well as toxicology journals, but as of this writing the FDA has not yet returned tryptophan to the dietary supplement market.

There is only one possible (although unacceptable) explanation for this—politics. Tryptophan is a safe and inexpensive competitor to a drug, and the FDA has had a long history of opposition to the therapeutic value of nutrients. Uncontaminated tryptophan is safe even by the FDA's own standards, since it is approved by the FDA for use in infant formulas, total intravenous feeding formulas, and in animal feed. The FDA's position toward dietary supplements has been successfully challenged, and I anticipate dramatic changes in their unduly harsh regulations, without any sacrifice of public safety. (For a more complete discussion on this topic, see Chapter 13.) Nonetheless, tryptophan is still unavailable except with a prescription.

Phenylalanine is available in two forms, DL-phenylalanine (DLPA) and L-phenylalanine (LPA). It appears that the DLPA is useful for the treatment of depression and is possibly helpful in chronic pain syndromes. Some depressed patients are more responsive to phenylalanine than to 5-hydroxytryptophan (5-HTP) because of differences in neurotransmitter abnormalities. It seems that some patients are depressed because of a lack of adequate norepinephrine, and they respond better to DL-phenylalanine than to 5-HTP.

How to Take Phenylalanine DL-phenylalanine is commonly available as 100- to 500-mg capsules. Typical doses are 250 to 1,500 mg of DLPA per day for depression. I suggest taking at least part of the dose at bedtime.

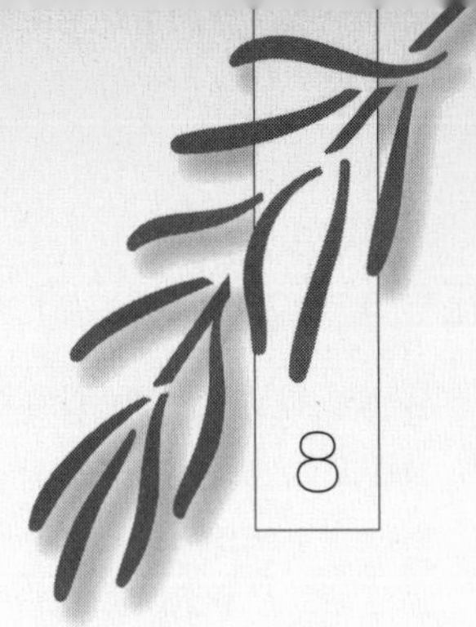

Flavonoids, Herbs, and Botanicals

A VARIETY OF PLANT-DERIVED SUPPLEMENTS have therapeutic and preventive properties for a number of health conditions. They fall into several categories, but as we learn more about the active components they are merging into one group. Herbs and botanicals contain flavonoids and other substances as their active principles. To some extent the distinction between herbs and botanicals is artificial. Different parts of the plants fall into one category or the other, but this is less important than knowing which ones help with what health problems.

Flavonoids

A wide variety of *phytochemicals* (plant chemicals) have powerful effects on physiological functions. Some of the newly discovered ones have had a lot of press recently as a result of their role in protecting against cancer and heart disease, as well as treating many other illnesses. (Of course, all vitamins are also phytochemicals, and well-known herbs also contain them; they are just not as newsworthy, as far as the press is concerned.)

The flavonoids (also called bioflavonoids) are phytochemical pigments that act as antioxidants to protect plants (and the animals that eat these plants—including you) from excess oxygen-free-radical damage. They enhance vitamin C activity and improve the strength of blood vessels, thus reducing bruising, bleeding gums, and the development of varicose veins and hemorrhoids. They also have a host of other physiological effects.

Various flavonoids help prevent cataract progression and macular degeneration, and they have been used to treat menopausal hot flashes. Bioflavonoids are also potent anti-inflammatory, antiallergic, anticancer, and antiviral agents. Some of the most recently available dietary supplements, such as quercetin, ginkgo extract, proanthocyanidins, and bilberry, contain substances in the bioflavonoid family. Some of the flavonoids are not yet available as supplements, once again calling attention to the importance of following a healthy, whole-foods diet.

Genistein is an "isoflavonoid," found in soy products and lima beans, that decreases the spread of tumors. It prevents the development of new blood vessels, reducing the supply of oxygen and nourishment to the tumor cells. Genistein also acts as a weak estrogen, blocking stronger estrogens from attaching to their receptor sites and preventing the stimulation that may give rise to cancer. Cultures with high soy intake have lower rates of breast and prostate cancers. Soy milk, tofu, tempeh, and miso are all good sources of genistein. It is available as a supplement as a component of several soy powders and in some capsules, but because soy foods are versatile and readily available, there is no real need for a supplement.

Herbs and Botanicals

In addition to those that contain flavonoids, there are many plant-derived supplements that come from various cultural heritages and healing arts throughout the ages. Many of our modern drugs were derived originally from herbal remedies. Digitalis, used in treating some forms of heart disease, comes from foxglove. Colchicine, a common treatment for gout, comes from colchicum, or autumn crocus. Some of the more potent medications for cancer come from common vinca plants, a perennial shrub also called periwinkle.

Most of the common herbs used in health care are very safe when used as directed, and far safer than almost any prescription medication, but it is valuable to have competent advice when using them for treatment, even if only for a proper diagnosis of the problem. Many certified nutritionists know how to use herbs in health care. There are some physicians who are knowledgeable about botanical remedies. Naturopathic physicians, or NDs (Doctors of Naturopathy), many chiropractors, and many M.D.'s who have sought special training all know quite a lot about this field. Most of the physicians who are members of the American College for Advancement in Medicine (ACAM) have knowledge of botanical medicines. Generally, the U.S. medical profession has been resistant to the use of herbal preparations, but this is gradually changing due to consumer demand and the increase in scientific studies supporting their use. Even the *Physician's Desk Reference* (*PDR*), the classic source of drug information, has come out with a *PDR for Herbal Medicines.*

There are many comprehensive treatises on herbs in health care, but this is not one of them. I do use a number of herbal preparations in practice, and they can be a valuable addition to your health care. Most of the time they are used for treatment of specific conditions, but some of them are used for general enhancement of physical performance, management of stress, support of endocrine glands, and increasing energy. For more thorough discussions of herbal remedies, see the books listed in Appendix 2.

Herbs are not orthomolecular substances. Unlike nutrients, they contain components that are not normally present in the body (but they also often contain nutrients). Although they are used for treatment and support of physiological processes, be aware that they are more likely than nutrients to have side effects when taken in high doses. The usual doses are quite safe, but you should not exceed them unless you are familiar with their use. I recommend standardized extracts of herbs when they are available. They are usually standardized to contain at least a specific amount of an active principle, which is also usually a marker for other active components. Standardization does not mean an extract that contains only the marker, but it has at least that amount of what is considered an important component. Much of the recent research on herbs has been done with standardized products.

Remember that natural, food- or plant-derived substances, such as herbs, flavonoids or botanicals, vary naturally in appearance from batch to batch depending on growing conditions and other influences. They may be darker or lighter, or have slightly different colors or textures. If you are concerned that something is really wrong with the ones you purchase, ask your source to confirm they are all right.

Mixed Bioflavonoids

There are many available supplements of mixed bioflavonoids, usually consisting of hesperidin, rutin, and citrus extracts. At one time the flavonoids were referred to as vitamin P, a term introduced by Albert Szent-Györgyi because they maintained normal permeability of membranes. They have antioxidant activity, and they enhance blood vessel strength, support the actions of vitamin C, and help in the treatment of hot flashes associated with menopause. Citrus bioflavonoids have been shown to protect tissues from the effects of radiation.

Sometimes bioflavonoids are mixed with vitamin C, and the combination is referred to as "vitamin C complex." However, it is usually less expensive and more flexible to take vitamin C and the bioflavonoids separately—you can then vary the doses independently. Bioflavonoids have general antioxidant effects and most have more specific, therapeutic benefits for health problems.

How to Take Mixed Bioflavonoids It is common to find mixed bioflavonoids in 500- to 1,000-mg tablets. I usually recommend 1,000 mg of mixed bioflavonoids twice a day for general antioxidant protection and blood vessel strength, especially for people who bruise easily. I also suggest this dose for help in the management of hot flashes associated with menopause and as part of a program for varicose veins.

Bilberry

Several species of blueberry (as well as other berries and cherries) contain compounds called anthocyanosides (similar to proanthocyanidins) that appear to have antioxidant properties and other therapeutic value. The European species of blueberry, found in Northern Europe, Asia, and North America, is called bilberry (*Vaccinium myrtillus*), and it has higher levels of these protective compounds.

Bilberry helps enhance vision and adaptation to the dark, and improves capillary circulation, which is especially important in the retina. It is also useful for diabetic visual impairment and for improving the health of the macula, the part of the retina where clearest vision takes place.

Loss of vision is the most feared disability. Visual deterioration is so common with advancing age, from cataracts, diabetes, hardening of the arteries, and age-related macular degeneration, that it is important to be careful with all health practices that may affect eyesight. Aside from the usual recommendations for diet and exercise, adding bilberry and other specific nutrient supplements is prudent for treatment and prevention.

How to Take Bilberry I have recommended bilberry extract as part of a comprehensive program for patients who have visual problems. Bilberry extract is available as a single ingredient, in 100-mg tablets or capsules. It is also frequently made as a combination of 100 mg of bilberry with other nutrients that protect the eye. It should say on the label that it is standardized to contain from 15 to 25 percent anthocyanosides. I usually recommend taking one capsule two or three times per day.

The combination that I use as vision nutrients contains 100 mg of the standardized bilberry extract, plus taurine, trace minerals, proanthocyanidins, ginkgo, and other antioxidants. Higher bilberry doses may help cataracts.

Black Cohosh

Black cohosh (*Cimicifuga racemosa*) has been used for menstrual and menopausal symptoms for centuries. In Germany it is now the most commonly used treatment for menopausal symptoms. Although it appears to attach to the cell receptors for estrogen, it is not clear that it actually has an estrogen effect, and the latest research suggests that this is unlikely. It may influence other female hormones to provide relief from hot flashes in menopause. The roots of the plant come off a "rhizome," which contains the active components of the herb.

The standardized herb contains 2.5 percent of a triterpene called deoxyacteine. Studies have shown that supplements of black cohosh can relieve not only hot flashes and night sweats, but also other symptoms related to menopause, such as depression, anxiety, insomnia, and loss of libido. In these effects it appears to be equal to taking estrogen hormone replacement therapy, although supplements of natural human estrogen (as opposed to Premarin from pregnant mares' urine) may have other benefits as well.

How to Take Black Cohosh Commonly available supplements of 40 mg of black cohosh extract that are standardized to 2.5 percent of 27-deoxyacteine will contain 1 mg of the active component. It is common to take 2 capsules twice a day for the complete relief of menopausal symptoms. When taken as part of a comprehensive program, it may be possible to take less and still have complete control of symptoms. I often recommend it with extra bioflavonoids, vitamin E, and isoflavones.

Cranberry

Cranberries contain several substances that are thought to be clinically effective in treatment of urinary tract infections (urethritis and cystitis). It is not clear which specific substances are the active components or exactly how they work, but both scientific studies and reports from many patients confirm the value of cranberry supplements in controlling cystitis and urethritis. (Cranberry also helps prevent the oxidation of the LDL cholesterol, and thus may play a role in protecting the heart and blood vessels.)

It is important to have a urine culture to diagnose urinary tract infections, and it may be essential to take the appropriate antibiotic for treatment. It is important not to let urinary infections go untreated because of the danger of developing a kidney infection. Cranberry may work by preventing bacteria from sticking to the bladder mucosal membrane.

Unfortunately, most commercial cranberry juice contains a large amount of sugar, and you have to drink quite a bit for it to be effective. Although such juices have been effective, these quantities of refined sugar are themselves detrimental to your immune system, making it more difficult to fight off infections. There is some unsweetened cranberry juice available at health food stores, but it is quite tart. If it is diluted with water and mixed with a small amount of fruit juice it can be palatable without enough sugar to adversely affect the immune system.

There are also capsules of cranberry powder available for supplemental use. These are what I usually recommend for urinary infections, in addition to extra vitamin C. (I also prescribe antibiotics as needed.)

How to Take Cranberry Cranberry powder is commonly available as 425-mg capsules. For most urinary infections, I suggest taking two capsules two or four times per day. If you are drinking the unsweetened juice, you may need up to one pint to be effective. This can be spread throughout the day. Sometimes a maintenance dose of cranberry supplements can prevent recurrence of infections.

Echinacea

Two herbal species, *Echinacea angustifolia* and *Echinacea purpurea*, are commonly used for enhancement of the immune system. They contain *echinacosides* and *sesquiterpenes*, which enhance white blood cell activity and increase interferon production. Echinacea increases both the number and activity of the white blood cells known as T-cells and the natural killer cells—which are essential to a healthy immune system. As is true of many herbs, very high doses may have side effects. However, the usual doses are generally quite safe.

Echinacea has antiviral and antibacterial activity, and it is useful in treating infections, although with serious bacterial infections I would also recommend the appropriate antibiotic. Echinacea has helped reduce the growth of herpes viruses, which cause genital herpes and cold sores (fever blisters). Because it stimulates white blood cells, echinacea may be helpful in supporting cancer treatments.

How to Take Echinacea Echinacea is available as capsules or tinctures, but the capsules are usually more convenient. Some people prefer the herbal tinctures diluted in water. Standardized echinacea capsules are available, and I now recommend a mixture containing 125 mg each of the angustifolia and purpurea varieties. This dose of 250 mg can be taken two to four times a day. It is usually best to take echinacea for a few weeks, and then stop for a week to avoid developing a tolerance to it. I take it occasionally, but if I feel a virus coming on I will take it consistently for a few days.

Feverfew

Feverfew (*Tanacetum parthenium*) has a long history of use for the treatment of fevers, headaches and joint inflammation. Active principles in feverfew are called *sesquiterpenes,* such as *parthenolide.* These inhibit prostaglandin production, leading to a reduction of inflammation. It is this anti-inflammatory property that may help treat arthritis. Feverfew also lowers histamine release.

Recent studies have documented the value of feverfew in the control of migraine headaches. As little as 25 mg twice per day has reduced both the intensity and the frequency of migraine headaches. It probably produces some of its effects as a result of alterations in serotonin production. Excess serotonin production by blood platelets can trigger constriction of the arteries. Migraines are possibly related to this constriction and subsequent relaxation of these blood vessels, but the mechanisms are not yet clear.

Some studies also report that feverfew reduces the excessive platelet stickiness that leads to blood clots inside the blood vessels. This is similar to the effects of garlic, ginkgo, and vitamin E. Thus it might be helpful in treating patients with heart disease in addition to its many other uses, although appropriate studies have not yet been done.

How to Take Feverfew Feverfew capsules are available in a variety of sizes. You can use the 380-mg capsules of freeze-dried leaves, but the level of the active components is quite variable, and the therapeutic value will vary with it. I usually recommend the standardized herbal extract, with a consistent 0.1 to 0.5 percent parthenolides. I suggest a 250-mg capsule twice per day as part of a program for the management of migraine headaches. The dose for helping arthritis has not been studied.

Garlic

Garlic (*Allium sativum*) has a long history of use in culinary arts, but it also has been used as a healing substance for centuries. It has been studied extensively in recent years, and the findings confirm many of its historical uses. Garlic reduces excessive blood clotting by decreasing platelet stickiness (platelets are small disk-shaped structures in the blood that initiate blood clots).

Garlic, as a food or a supplement, lowers cholesterol and blood pressure and helps to kill yeast in the intestinal tract. It contains sulfur compounds (allylic sulfides), including allicin and alliin, that help to detoxify many carcinogens and protect you from developing cancer. It is also being studied for the treatment of cancer.

Many different garlic preparations are on the market, and they are being highly publicized. The most potent preparations are the "deodorized" forms (not "odorless," which is also sold), which contain the equivalent of many cloves of garlic in each pill. The substances that produce the odor in garlic are excreted by the lungs, leading to "garlic breath," and they also come out through the pores of the skin, which is why many people prefer the deodorized preparations. According to some researchers, each of the brands that they used in their studies was effective in producing experimental responses, although there was some variation. When garlic is crushed, alliin is converted to allicin, but the enzyme that does this conversion is destroyed by heat. The conversion will take place if the garlic is allowed to stand after crushing, for ten minutes before the cooking starts.

How to Take Garlic Deodorized garlic powder is commonly available in 350- to 500-mg capsules. I usually suggest taking one or two of the 500-mg capsules twice per day. It is also available as a liquid, but this is not as convenient as the capsules. In case you are wondering, the deodorized brands do not leave you with "garlic breath."

Ginger

Ginger (*Zingiber officinale*) has a long history of medicinal and culinary use originally in southeast Asia, and now virtually everywhere else. In addition to its wonderful flavor, it contains antioxidants, pungent substances, and aromatic oils that have therapeutic properties. Ginger has been shown to help with nausea due to motion sickness or morning sickness (nausea and vomiting of pregnancy) more effectively than common medications. It is also useful for reducing excessive blood clotting in heart patients and lowering cholesterol and triglycerides.

The active compounds in ginger include gingerol, shogaol, and zingerone. Recently studies have confirmed that standardized extracts of ginger containing gingerol can reduce tumor growth and inhibit inflammation. The anti-inflammatory effects of ginger powder have been shown to relieve arthritis symptoms in patients with rheumatoid or osteoarthritis. Another effect of ginger is to increase the strength of the heart muscle. This might help with congestive heart failure, but so far I have seen no clinical studies that examine this.

How to Take Ginger It is a pleasure to take ginger as a flavoring for foods, and indeed this is effective for many of the benefits that it can provide. It is also effective either as a tea (made by boiling ginger root in water), or by adding minced ginger or powdered ginger to cooked dishes. Effective doses are from 2 to 4 grams per day of the powdered herb. As a supplement, ginger is available as a standardized extract, containing 5 percent of the pungent compounds (gingerol and shogaol) or 4 percent of the volatile oils. Typical doses are 250 to 500 mg twice a day for arthritis or morning sickness.

Ginkgo Biloba

Ginkgo biloba extract comes from the leaf of the ancient tree of the same name. The extract contains terpene substances, known as ginkgolides and bilobalides, which improve circulation to the brain in patients with hardening of the arteries. This increases the oxygen supply and availability of other nutrients to the brain and results in generally improved central nervous system function. It has been shown in scientific studies to improve memory, especially short-term memory, to enhance concentration, and to relieve associated depression.

Ginkgo also contains a variety of bioflavonoids that act as free-radical scavengers and antioxidants. In addition to these nonspecific benefits and memory enhancement, ginkgo extract helps with peripheral vascular disease, vertigo (dizziness), tinnitus (ringing in the ears), migraine headaches, and Raynaud's phenomenon (spasms in the blood vessels of the hands or feet, usually brought on by exposure to cold). Because degenerative eye diseases, such as macular degeneration, are probably related to oxidation and poor microcirculation, ginkgo has been suggested for these conditions.

Most of the scientific studies on Ginkgo biloba have been done with a 24 percent standardized extract, not the plain powdered leaf. Capsules of the powdered leaf are also available, but the level of active components is not as consistent as in the standardized product.

How to Take Ginkgo Biloba Capsules of the 24 percent standardized *Ginkgo biloba* extract are available in 40- to 60-mg sizes. I usually recommend taking about 120 mg per day (two or three capsules depending on the size), although I have sometimes recommended higher doses for more severe vascular disease or for patients with memory loss who do not respond to the lower doses.

Ginseng

Several varieties of ginseng are prized for their health-enhancing properties. American and Korean ginsengs (*Panax quinquefolium* and *Panax ginseng*, respectively), and Siberian ginseng (*Eleutherococcus senticosus*, not a true ginseng, but with some similar effects) are somewhat different in their properties, but they are all known as "adaptogens," or substances that help the body adapt to stresses of different kinds. The active compounds in the American and Korean ginsengs are *ginsenosides, saponins,* and *phytosterols.* Usually the American ginseng is considered more relaxing and the Korean more stimulating, but both can enhance energy and stamina. Standardized extracts of these ginsengs contain 15 percent ginsenosides.

Ginseng can protect the heart muscle and the lining cells of the arteries from oxidative damage, and protect cells against the effects of radiation. It may also enhance the improvements in male sexual function that result from taking the amino acid arginine, because it increases the release of nitric oxide, essential for normal erections with sexual stimulation. Ginseng supplements can decrease allergic responses and inflammation and enhance learning and memory. A number of studies show that it can also inhibit initiation and growth of malignant tumors.

Siberian ginseng contains eleutherosides that appear to help the adrenal glands respond to stress. It may enhance stamina and reduce fatigue. It helps to resist infections and stimulate immune function. Standardized extracts contain 0.8 percent eleutherosides.

How to Take Ginseng Ginseng is available in many forms, from powdered roots to tinctures to standardized extracts. The average dose of the root is 2 to 4 grams a day. The usual doses of standardized ginseng extracts range from 200 to 400 mg twice a day. Capsules of 100 to 200 mg of standardized extract are available. You can take ginseng daily for specific conditions or as needed in times of stress or fatigue as a supplement to the rest of your health program.

Possible side effects from these stimulant herbs include nervousness, insomnia, and irritability. If you experience these, reduce the dose or stop taking the herb.

Grapefruit Seed Extract

Substances in grapefruit and other citrus seeds have strong antifungal properties. That is, they kill yeast (fungus), often better than the medications used for the same purpose (for example, Nystatin). Since many people have an overgrowth of the yeasts that are normally present in the intestinal tract, grapefruit seed extract is often helpful with a variety of symptoms. These symptoms are related to what is known as chronic candidiasis, which is *not* an infection, but an *overgrowth.*

Remember, these yeasts (or *Candida albicans*) are normally in your intestines, although as yet we do not know if they perform any useful functions. They do compete with the known friendly bacteria, such as *Lactobacillus acidophilus* and *Bifidobacterium bifidum*.

The overabundant intestinal yeasts release many toxins (called *mycotoxins*), which may give you a variety of systemic symptoms, including headaches, fatigue, depression, and poor immune function. Overabundance of yeast also causes recurrent vaginal yeast infections and digestive disturbances. These symptoms occur even though the yeasts do *not* leave the intestines to colonize other tissues, although the recurrent vaginal yeast infections are due to the migration of yeasts from the anal area. This distinction has confused many patients and has led many physicians to dismiss intestinal yeasts as a cause of systemic symptoms. Serious systemic yeast *infections* do occur in debilitated patients with severe immune dysfunction, cancer, or other systemic diseases—but this is a different situation requiring much more vigorous medical treatment.

How to Take Grapefruit Seed Extract Grapefruit seed extract is available as a liquid or in capsules containing powder. The liquid is awkward and has a strong taste, and it must be diluted to prevent local irritation of the mucous membranes. A few drops in a glass of water is still quite a strong preparation.

I recommend the capsules for convenience and to avoid any local mucous membrane irritation. It is available in 100-mg capsules, and usually one or two capsules twice daily is sufficient. Sometimes a third dose is helpful for resistant yeast-related symptoms.

Guggulipids

Guggulipids are resins derived from guggulow, an extract from the guggul tree (*Commiphora mukul*), which grows only in particular areas of India. It has a long folk history in Ayurvedic medicine. Recent scientific evidence shows that the lipid sterols called guggulsterones that it contains can lower total serum cholesterol levels while increasing the level of good HDL cholesterol.

It is not clear how it works, although guggulipids do have antioxidant effects that may account for some of its benefits, and the resins may bind with cholesterol in the intestinal tract preventing their reabsorption. Some of my patients have seen their high cholesterol levels come down and their HDL levels go up in response to supplements of this botanical even when they have not made the recommended dietary changes. It also has been shown to help with cystic acne, and it has demonstrated anti-inflammatory effects in laboratory animals who were given injections of chemicals to produce arthritis.

How to Take Guggulipids There are capsules of guggulow containing 340 mg of plant extract with 0.4 percent essential oils. There are also capsules of 250 mg guggulipid standardized extracts, containing 2.5 percent of the *guggulsterones.* For management of high cholesterol levels, the typical doses range from 250 to 500 mg of the standardized extract twice a day as part of a comprehensive lipid-lowering program.

Hawthorn Berry

Hawthorn (*Crataegus oxycantha*) is a large shrub or small tree that you may see growing in many areas. It produces small red berries that contain a number of anthocyanidins and other flavonoids. Research shows that supplements of hawthorn berry extract can lower blood pressure by dilating blood vessels, improve the cardiovascular function of patients with congestive heart failure, and reduce angina.

Hawthorn also has many of the other properties of anthocyanidin flavonoids, such as reducing allergy reactions and improving the strength of capillaries. Because of the dilation of blood vessels, it may help with Raynaud's phenomenon (spasms of the blood vessels in the hands). Much of the recent research has been done using standardized extracts, containing at least 2 percent of vitexin, one of the active compounds.

How to Take Hawthorn Berry Capsules containing standardized extract of hawthorn berry (2 percent standard) usually contain 100 to 250 mg of extract. Typical doses for congestive heart failure would be 250 mg, twice per day. The same dose range would be helpful for high blood pressure. You must take it consistently for a period of at least a few weeks for these benefits. Higher doses are sometimes recommended, but when comprehensive health promotion programs are initiated, and other effective supplements are included, it is often unnecessary to use the higher level of any one supplement.

Kava Kava

This Polynesian herb (also known simply as kava) is traditionally used as a beverage for its psychoactive effects and as a calming agent because of its antianxiety properties. It contains a group of substances collectively called kavalactones (or kava pyrones), which have a relaxant effect and appear to produce a mild sense of euphoria. Although some antianxiety drugs may induce depression, fatigue, or reduced mental clarity and memory, kava has no such side effects. If you are taking these medications, most physicians advise gradually stopping them before introducing kava as an alternative, as it may increase the effects of these antianxiety drugs. Long-term, heavy usage of the herb has been known to cause a scaly skin rash, but this is not seen with typical doses.

Unlike the conventional medications for anxiety (Valium, Xanax, Serax, and others in the benzodiazapine group), kava is not addictive and it does not become less effective when taken over a period of time. However, if anxiety is persistent, it is best to try to find the cause rather than only taking substances that can help relieve the symptoms. Aside from anxiety-provoking life situations, it is common for low blood sugar (or hypoglycemia), food allergies, candidiasis, and other conditions to produce anxiety. If you are taking kava regularly for anxiety or to help you sleep, it is best to limit its use to four or five months and then take a break. The reason to stop taking kava kava after several months is that it seems to be more effective with periodic breaks.

How to Take Kava Kava Standardized extract of kava, with 30 percent of the kavalactones, is available in 150- to 250-mg capsules. It is common to take two or three of these capsules a day to relieve anxiety and help promote restful sleep. You might find that just one pill at night is enough, but you can take two or three spread throughout the day. The benefits tend to increase with time, even up to six months, so give kava some time to work.

Licorice Extract (DGL)

This is an extract of licorice (*Glycyrrhiza glabra*) that has had the *glycyrrhizin* removed. Glycyrrhizin is a component of licorice with some possible toxicity, although it has antiviral activity and some other therapeutic uses. At high doses, the glycyrrhizin may cause elevation of blood pressure due to its hormonelike effects.

The deglycyrrhizinated licorice (you can see why it is called DGL) is activated when chewed well and mixed with saliva. It then coats the esophagus and stomach, forming a protective layer against stomach acid. It can relieve the symptoms of hiatal hernia, gastritis, gastroesophageal reflux disorder (GERD), and ulcers, thus letting the tissues heal, without the need for antacids or antihistamine drugs such as Zantac or Prilosec. Comparative studies show that DGL is as good as the antihistamine drugs for the treatment of stomach and duodenal ulcers.

The real problem with peptic ulcers is not usually too much acid in the stomach, but rather an increased sensitivity of the lining cells to normal levels of acid. There is also reason to suspect that a refined-food diet, with low fiber and plenty of sugar, and coffee and alcohol consumption contribute to the causation of ulcer disease, as do high stress levels.

Current information shows that there is a bacterium, called *Helicobacter pylori*, which causes most ulcers. Interestingly, this bacterium grows better when there is less acid in the stomach. This would suggest that all the antihistamine drugs (which block stomach acid production) and antacids that people take may actually increase their risk of developing ulcers. The antihistamine drugs are among the most frequently prescribed medications.

How to Take Licorice Extract DGL is available as chewable tablets that taste strongly of licorice. Even if you do not like the flavor of licorice, the benefits to your digestive system will probably keep you taking this supplement. Most of the DGL supplements on the market contain a small amount of fructose (extracted fruit sugar) to make the licorice flavor palatable, but it is also available without sweetener.

For best results, chew one or two tablets of DGL before each meal, or take one or two any time that you feel symptoms of acid indigestion.

Proanthocyanidins

Proanthocyanidin (PAC) bioflavonoids (also called procyanidolic oligomers) are powerful antioxidants and free-radical scavengers. A number of physiological and nutritional substances appear to have difficulty getting into the brain tissue, which has led scientists to surmise that there is a physiological barrier, not an actual physical wall, protecting the brain. Proanthocyanidins, however, do cross this so-called blood-brain barrier, which allows them to act as antioxidants in the brain. The brain is largely made up of fatty tissue that is prone to oxidative damage.

Proanthocyanidins are helpful in slowing the aging process, improving blood vessel and connective tissue strength, and detoxifying the body. They often help with allergies and as anti-inflammatory agents. PACs may reduce the risk of cancer, heart disease, and stroke, and reduce the inflammation in arthritis.

The PACs are natural plant products, which were first studied as supplements derived from the bark of a European pine tree (the Pycnogenol brand). These compounds and other related substances are also found in grape seed extracts, which are now available as supplements. Most of the research by the originator, Dr. Jacques Masquelier, has been done with the grape seed extract. It is also cheaper than the pine bark extract.

The latest information is that the grape seed extract is an even better source of active product, although there are compounds present in each source that are not present in the other. Proanthocyanidins act within cell membranes, and they neutralize both water- and fat-soluble free radicals. They also inhibit the release of enzymes that damage capillaries. Proanthocyanidins have been shown to be safe in numerous tests over many years.

How to Take Proanthocyanidins Both grape seed and pine bark extracts are available individually or as mixtures. I usually recommend a 50-mg capsule twice per day of a mixture containing 40 mg of grape seed extract and 10 mg of pine bark extract. Sometimes people start with higher doses and then taper down to 50 to 100 mg per day.

Quercetin

This brilliant yellow-green bioflavonoid has a special effect on certain cell membranes. It has an affinity for the cells that release histamine and serotonin, the mediators of the allergic and inflammatory responses. It stabilizes the membranes of these *mast cells* and *basophils*, reducing their chemical release. These membranes are often leaky in allergy sufferers, allowing excessive release of the allergy mediators. Quercetin can also help asthma patients, reducing their sensitivity to allergens. Interestingly, a drug with a similar effect, cromolyn, is a synthetic flavonoid.

Quercetin reduces the activity of an enzyme aldose reductase. This in turn decreases the deposition of sugar-protein complexes in the lens of the eye, and lowers your risk of developing cataracts. Limiting sugar intake is also helpful with cataract prevention, especially the milk sugar lactose, because of the effect of one of its components—galactose—on increasing cataract formation. Another effect of quercetin is to reduce the damage induced by tobacco smoke in the airway membranes. Even if you do not smoke yourself, it is hard to completely avoid exposure to secondhand smoke so quercetin may also benefit nonsmokers.

How to Take Quercetin I usually suggest doses of 400 mg of quercetin twice per day for allergic patients and those at risk of cataracts. Sometimes they need to increase the dose to 1,200 or 1,600 mg per day for asthma or more severe allergy symptoms. The product I use contains 400 mg of quercetin, mixed with the enzyme bromelain to help enhance its absorption.

Saw Palmetto

The saw palmetto tree (*Serenoa repens*) is a small palm tree that produces reddish-brown berries that are therapeutic for prostate gland enlargement. The prostate gland is the male organ (about the size of a walnut) located under the bladder and surrounding the neck of the bladder and the urine outflow channel—the urethra. Certain fat-soluble substances in the berries (saponins and phytosterols) help to reduce benign enlargement of the prostate, and this relieves abnormal pressure on the urethra.

Benign enlargement of the prostate is very common in men over forty. A recently developed drug, finasteride (Proscar), may also help the prostate, but it has side effects and it is not as effective as the saw palmetto extract, which is safer. (The FDA sees fit to allow medical claims for the drug, but not for the herbal extract.) Saw palmetto is part of a comprehensive approach to the treatment of prostate enlargement.

Symptoms of prostate enlargement are difficulty starting urination, slow urine flow, frequent urination, urgency, retained urine in the bladder, dripping after completion of urination, and nighttime urination interrupting sleep. Saw palmetto extract helps all these symptoms, possibly by interfering with the production of a testosterone metabolite called dihydrotestosterone that is a strong stimulant of prostate enlargement.

How to Take Saw Palmetto Saw palmetto is available as 120- to 160-mg capsules. The usual therapeutic level is 300 to 500 mg per day. I recommend the 160-mg capsules taken twice per day, and an additional capsule if the symptoms are not responding or are particularly severe. The alternative is to take a less effective medication or to wait until the symptoms are severe enough to require surgical reduction of prostate tissue.

Two other herbs also benefit the symptoms of prostate enlargement. Combining *Pygeum africanum* and *Urtica dioica* (stinging nettle) with saw palmetto is helpful with the symptoms more than the individual supplements separately. They reduce the irritation and sensitivity of the bladder and urethra, thus reducing the symptoms of frequency and urgency. The typical doses are 25 mg of Pygeum and 125 mg of stinging nettle, each taken twice per day. I like to combine the three nutrients, and there are also preparations that incorporate them with zinc and beneficial amino acids and essential fatty acids.

Silymarin (Milk Thistle Extract)

Silymarin is a combination of several components extracted from milk thistle (*Silybum marianum*). These are flavonoid antioxidants with specific benefits for the liver. They aid in the healing of already damaged liver, and they protect the liver from the damaging effects of environmental chemicals. As with other flavonoids, some of the benefits are the result of reduced cell-membrane damage induced by free radicals. Silymarin also improves sugar levels in diabetics and reduces their urinary sugar spillover. It reduces capillary fragility and excess blood vessel permeability. Silymarin is also valuable in helping to reduce cholesterol levels.

Silymarin probably produces some of its clinical effects by restoring liver cell membranes and by increasing the sensitivity of insulin receptors. As a result, diabetics may be able to safely decrease their insulin doses. (Do not do so without medical supervision.) Interestingly, silymarin is used to treat liver diseases in many countries other than the United States, but the U.S. physician resistance to botanical medicine is gradually changing.

How to Take Silymarin Supplements of milk thistle extract, standardized with 80 percent silymarin, are available in 150-mg capsules. Two capsules twice per day is an effective dose for liver protection and sugar improvement. For general protection, one or two capsules per day may be adequate, unless you are highly exposed to damaging environmental chemicals.

St. John's Wort

St. John's wort (also called *Hypericum perforatum* or simply hypericum) is useful in the treatment of depression and anxiety, as well as insomnia. Although it has some properties similar to the drugs known as "selective serotonin reuptake inhibitors" or SSRIs, such as Prozac and Zoloft, and other antidepressant drugs called MAO inhibitors, it does not have serious side effects. When taken in the typical doses, even mild side effects are unusual (digestive upset and dizziness). Scientific studies show that St. John's wort is as effective as the drugs for mild to moderately severe depression. Higher doses may help more severe depression.

Be cautious about taking St. John's wort with MAO inhibitor drugs. It is possible to switch from the SSRI drugs to the herb in the treatment of depression and anxiety, but it is best to do so with medical supervision, gradually reducing the dose of the medication and increasing the herb over a few weeks. In animals and possibly also in humans, St. John's wort can cause sensitivity to ultraviolet light (photosensitivity), so it is best to stay out of excessive sunlight while taking the herb, or else wear adequate clothing for protection.

St. John's wort contains many active components including flavonoids and terpenes, but the standardized herb contains a minimum amount of hypericin (0.3 to 0.5 percent), one of the chemicals that appear to have therapeutic properties. These chemicals appear to affect the levels of several different neurotransmitters, which is likely how St. John's wort reduces depression and anxiety.

How to Take St. John's Wort St. John's wort is typically available in tinctures, tablets, or capsules. I recommend capsules of the standardized extract. Typical doses are 300 mg of the standardized extract (at least 0.3 percent hypericin) taken three times a day. It takes some time for the effect of St. John's wort to develop, so give it at least a few weeks' trial.

Depression and anxiety are complex issues, and it is best to take St. John's wort as part of a comprehensive program that includes stress reduction and exercise, as well as a sugar-free diet. Counseling may also be an important part of a total program.

Stinging Nettle (Urtica dioica)

The stinging nettle plant (*Urtica dioica*), also called common nettle, has little surface hairs that release a stinging acid when touched. This property is lost in cooking or in processing to make supplements. The plant extract is used therapeutically as a diuretic and for its properties in relieving allergies and hay fever symptoms. It is also used for anti-inflammatory effects, which help with arthritis.

Stinging nettle has a number of active components including flavonoids, silica, and volatile oils, as well as some neurotransmitters that may contribute to its therapeutic properties. It also contains some sterols and lectins. Recent studies have incorporated nettle into regimens for treatment of prostate enlargement, not because it shrinks the prostate, but because it relieves the urethral and bladder irritation that increases urgency and frequency. It is also used for urinary tract infections.

How to Take Stinging Nettle The amount of nettle used for prostate enlargement ranges from 250 to 750 mg per day. The same dose would be the amount for treatment of arthritic symptoms or as a diuretic. Doses from 250 to 500 mg several times a day are common for allergic symptoms such as hay fever, taken as needed when the symptoms occur.

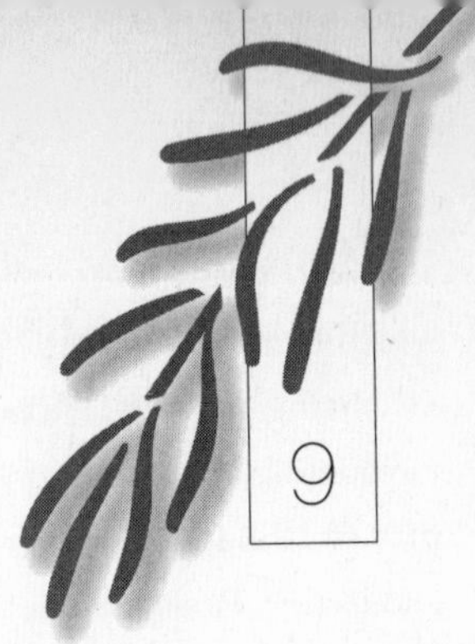

9

Accessory Supplements

ACCESSORY SUPPLEMENTS are those dietary supplements that do not readily fit into other categories of nutritional supplements. They include nonessential nutrients that may become essential in certain situations, as well as hormones or tissue components that are valuable as supplements for certain conditions, especially as people age.

These supplements include calcium D-glucarate, coenzyme Q_{10}, DHEA, glucosamine sulfate, ipriflavone, lactobacilli and other intestinal flora, lipoic acid, melatonin, methylsulfonylmethane (MSM), and phosphatidyl serine. (L-carnitine is not a true amino acid, but it is so closely related to them that I included it in chapter 7.)

Calcium D-Glucarate

Calcium D-glucarate is a safe, natural compound that is produced in small amounts in the body. It is present in all cells and in some vegetables and fruits. It is especially important for the organs of detoxification, such as the liver, spleen, and kidneys, and for the intestinal lining, breast, and endocrine glands. It is converted in the body into a potent cancer protective compound called D-glucaro-1,4-lactone. Many toxins and carcinogens such as pesticides, PCBs, hydrocarbons, and drugs are eliminated by attachment to a substance called glucuronic acid. An enzyme called beta-glucuronidase blocks this detoxification, but D-glucaro-1,4-lactone counteracts this enzyme, thus facilitating elimination of the chemicals.

If toxins and used hormones are not broken down, they then promote tumor formation and tumor progression. Calcium D-glucarate is unlike most anticancer supplements in that its activity against cancer is not related to antioxidant activity, but to this influence on enzymes. As a supplement it is used in general detoxification health programs.

The main research on calcium D-glucarate is in animals, in which it inhibits a variety of tumors, but it is such a safe compound that it is a good idea to include it in any cancer treatment program, and also for people who are at increased risk of developing cancer.

How to Take Calcium D-Glucarate Calcium D-glucarate is commonly available in 500-mg capsules. For general detoxification, I recommend taking from one to three capsules a day. For patients with cancer, I usually recommend going much higher, up to six to nine capsules a day. If you are exposed to environmental toxins, it is a good idea to take calcium D-glucarate to help eliminate them before they can do their damage. In these situations, you might take three to six capsules a day for a few weeks or a few months.

Coenzyme Q_{10}

Coenzyme Q_{10} (CoQ_{10}) is not a vitamin, but it is a fat-soluble antioxidant nutrient that is normally produced in the body. It is sometimes called ubiquinone. There are circumstances in which your own production of coenzyme Q_{10} is inadequate for optimal health, and it becomes a "conditionally essential" nutrient. CoQ_{10} is essential for the production of ATP (adenosine triphosphate) in the little cellular engines called mitochondria. ATP is the molecule that our cells use to store energy.

With both age and illness, the production of CoQ_{10} declines. Especially after the age of forty, our tissue levels of CoQ_{10} are markedly lower. Supplements can prevent and treat a variety of conditions, including heart disease, hypertension, rheumatic valvular disease, and arrhythmias. Coenzyme Q_{10} supplements reduce angina (heart pain) and increase exercise tolerance. In people with congestive heart failure, it can improve the strength of the heart muscle and reduce shortness of breath. Some patients who had been told by their doctors that they needed a heart transplant because of the severity of their heart disease have improved so dramatically with CoQ_{10} supplements that they have been able to avoid surgery and to resume many of their normal activities.

Coenzyme Q_{10} also stimulates normal immune function, and it helps people with chronic fatigue syndrome and other immune system disorders. It reduces inflammation of the gums (gingivitis)—one of its earliest described therapeutic uses. CoQ_{10} stabilizes cell membranes, improves sugar metabolism in diabetics, improves metabolic rate, and slows the aging process. Because of the combination of antioxidant activity and immune support, coenzyme Q_{10} may be very helpful in patients with multiple allergies and environmental illness.

Like a number of other nutrients, coenzyme Q_{10} helps so many problems, it sometimes seems like a miracle cure. This appears to be the case only when one does not understand the physiology behind its many real health benefits.

How to Take Coenzyme Q_{10} The usual therapeutically effective dose of coenzyme Q_{10} is 50 to 200 mg per day, although higher doses are often helpful in more severe heart disease. Recent reports suggest that those higher doses (200 to 600 mg) may also aid in the treatment of cancer, immune dysfunction, chronic fatigue syndrome, and severe congestive heart failure. It is clear that supplements significantly increase the blood and tissue levels of coenzyme Q_{10}.

Although CoQ_{10} is fat soluble, it is not toxic and does not accumulate excessively in the tissues. It is important to take it with food or in a chewable tablet containing some oils for best absorption. It is usually available in capsules containing 30 to 50 mg, or in chewable tablets that contain up to 100 to 200 mg of CoQ_{10}, usually mixed with some lecithin to enhance absorption. There is chewable CoQ_{10} on the market containing some synthetic vitamin E in the base. Although synthetic vitamin E is not harmful and does have antioxidant value, I prefer the natural form. A gel-based coenzyme Q_{10} is available, and it is better absorbed than the other forms, but it is usually significantly more expensive than the chewable tablets.

I usually recommend 100 to 200 mg per day for people who have immune system disorders or fatigue, or for anyone over forty years old, when production of CoQ_{10} is significantly lower. If they have heart problems or cancer, I usually use the higher doses, ranging from 200 to 400 mg per day, and sometimes even more.

DHEA (Dehydroepiandrosterone)

DHEA is a steroid hormone that is manufactured in the adrenal glands and is the precursor to other hormones, including testosterone, progesterone and other estrogens, and corticosterone. The adrenal produces more DHEA than any other hormone, and it has been referred to as the "mother" hormone. DHEA influences many physiological functions in the body, including energy, mood, memory, blood pressure, infections and immunity, tumor growth, sugar regulation, and weight. Blood levels of DHEA steadily decline with age, and this decline is considered one of the biological markers of aging. Many physicians measure the level of DHEA-S (the sulfate metabolite of DHEA) in the blood to evaluate the need for supplements.

Supplements of DHEA that reverse the age-related decline in blood levels may help to treat or prevent heart disease, cancer, diabetes, obesity, Alzheimer's disease, and immune disorders, such as rheumatoid arthritis. When levels are low, there appears to be greater risk of these conditions. DHEA also may help with osteoporosis, either by directly increasing levels of estrogens and testosterone, or by an indirect elevation of progesterone levels. Some physicians are recommending DHEA simply to help slow down or reverse the aging process. Although formerly available only by prescription, DHEA is now available as a dietary supplement. I recommend a blood level determination before supplementing with DHEA, because, although it has a remarkable safety profile, when dealing with hormones it is good to maintain some level of caution.

How to Take DHEA Typical doses of DHEA range from 5 mg per day up to 100 mg or more. The sublingual (under-the-tongue) form is thought by some to be better because it is dissolved in the mouth and therefore not digested before delivery into the bloodstream. With sublingual doses it is common to use 5 to 25 mg per day. It is wise to have blood levels checked periodically while on DHEA to make sure it is in the appropriate range. Many physicians feel that you should try to restore your level to that of someone in the twenty-to-thirty-year-old age range, as these are the levels associated with prevention of the above conditions.

Glucosamine Sulfate

Glucosamine sulfate is not really a vitamin, but it is the major amino sugar in the body. It is formed from glucose using the amino acid glutamine as the source of the amino group. Amino sugars are important components of connective tissue, including cartilage, the rubbery material in the joints that protects them from wear and tear.

When joints are inflamed from osteoarthritis (degenerative joint disease), supplements of glucosamine sulfate are often helpful in relieving symptoms and restoring joint integrity. Glucosamine sulfate actually stimulates new cartilage formation to protect the bone surface. In fact, studies have shown that taking glucosamine sulfate is better than the usual drugs for arthritis, called nonsteroidal anti-inflammatory drugs (or NSAIDs), like Motrin, Indocin, Advil, and Naprosyn.

With NSAIDs treatment, the joints are not helped, but the symptoms are frequently relieved—as long as you keep taking the drugs. These drugs have side effects, including ulcers and gastrointestinal bleeding, and beneath the pain relief, the joint destruction continues. Glucosamine sulfate does not have side effects, and after taking it for three to six weeks, it actually reduces symptoms better than the NSAIDs.

Chondroitin sulfate is another supplement that has recently been shown to be helpful in osteoarthritis. Although it is a large molecule and only about 12 percent of that taken orally is absorbed, it helps to reduce both inflammation and symptoms in a number of studies. It is not clear that there is any benefit to taking it in addition to glucosamine sulfate, but the current research supports both substances.

How to Take Glucosamine Sulfate Glucosamine sulfate is usually available as 500-mg capsules, and the usual effective dose is three or four capsules daily. I usually recommend two capsules twice per day. If the situation is more severe, six capsules may be necessary to achieve results. Newly available forms, such as *N*-acetyl glucosamine and glucosamine HCl, have not been proven effective. They have no apparent advantages over glucosamine sulfate.

Chondroitin sulfate is usually beneficial at a dose of 1,200 mg per day. It appears to make no difference whether it is taken in one dose or divided into three a day.

Ipriflavone

Ipriflavone is a relative of the isoflavones found in food sources such as soybean products. Its chemical name is isopropoxy isoflavone, and although very small amounts are found in food, the major source for supplements is synthetic. The soy isoflavones appear to help prevent or even treat cancer and heart disease. It is very likely that large amounts of soy products in the diet (tofu, tempeh, soymilk, toasted soynuts, and soy protein powders) or as supplements will also help prevent or reverse osteoporosis (thinning of the bones with age), but so far the research is limited. On the other hand, research is strongly supportive of a role for ipriflavone not only in retarding osteoporosis, but also in increasing bone density in patients who already have osteoporosis.

Ipriflavone can reduce the need for estrogen replacement therapy when it is being used to retard bone loss. However, it can also be part of a comprehensive program including natural human estrogens and progesterone as well as diet, exercise, and other supplements. Studies on ipriflavone have come from Italy, Japan, and Hungary where it is used extensively for bone health. It can increase bone density between 3 and 9 percent in as little as six months to a year. This is a very significant increase in bone density.

Although isoflavones from soybeans and other sources may relieve or diminish many menopausal symptoms, such as hot flashes, depression, irritability, and insomnia, so far no studies show that ipriflavone has the same effects.

How to Take Ipriflavone The effective dose of ipriflavone for osteoporosis is 600 mg per day. The capsules usually come in 200- to 300-mg sizes, and most of the research is done with 200 mg three times a day. However, it is very likely that taking 300 mg twice a day will be just as effective, and it is much more likely that you will remember to take them if you only have to do it twice a day.

I commonly recommend 300 mg twice a day because it is more convenient and less expensive. So far, no research suggests that higher doses will be more helpful. Ipriflavone is a useful and safe alternative to estrogen replacement therapy for purposes of increasing bone density.

Lactobacilli

Lactobacilli are often referred to as the "friendly bacteria" found in the normal digestive tract. They have many health benefits that go beyond improving digestion. These are the bacteria that are present in yogurts *if* they contain live cultures, which should be clearly stated on the label. If the label says "made with live cultures," it does not say whether they were killed by pasteurization *after* the yogurt was made.

The most common cause for reduction of intestinal flora is antibiotic treatments. Antibiotics are often given for repeated infections or even for the treatment of acne. Antibiotic use can lead to diarrhea. If antibiotic treatment is necessary, it is wise to take some replacement flora after the treatment is finished. The usual supplements of intestinal flora contain *Lactobacillus acidophilus* and *Bifidobacterium bifidum.* Other intestinal bacteria are available, but these appear to be the most important.

The normal flora maintain healthy intestinal function, and they also produce some vitamins, including vitamin K and some B vitamins. Supplements of lactobacilli and bifidobacteria help treat both constipation and diarrhea, including traveler's diarrhea, and they help manage both irritable colon and ulcerative colitis, as well as Crohn's disease. In addition, they have antifungal, antibacterial, and antiviral properties. These bacteria also produce some anticancer substances, helping both to degrade some carcinogens and reduce the growth of other bacteria that may promote cancer.

The vaginal flora of healthy women are predominantly lactobacilli. Supplements of lactobacilli can prevent and treat vaginal, urinary tract, and intestinal infections. These supplements may also be given intravaginally. Recurrent vaginal yeast infections are often helped by treating the overgrowth of yeast in the intestinal tract.

How to Take Lactobacilli Intestinal flora supplements come in both powder and capsule forms. The potent forms should contain at least ten billion organisms per gram. Typical doses are ⅓ to ½ teaspoon of the powder twice daily. For capsules, the usual dose is one or two capsules twice daily. Occasionally, some people report increased diarrhea from too much friendly flora supplementation.

Lipoic Acid

Lipoic acid (also called alpha-lipoic acid or thioctic acid) is a sulfur-containing, vitaminlike substance that is not usually essential in the diet as it is manufactured in the body. It may be essential in certain situations, and in high doses it is therapeutic for certain conditions. Lipoic acid is an antioxidant that helps control free radicals in both water and fat components of the cells. It is effective both inside and outside the cells.

In diabetics, lipoic acid has been shown to help control blood sugar and treat the neuropathy that often develops. Neuropathy can occur in many tissues and organs, but it most commonly starts in the legs. Symptoms of peripheral neuropathy are numbness and tingling, or pins-and-needles sensations, increased nerve sensitivity, and pain in the legs and feet. Lipoic acid can help when the nerves to the heart are damaged (cardiac autonomic neuropathy) as is sometimes seen in diabetics.

Lipoic acid may increase levels of the antioxidant glutathione as well as coenzyme Q_{10} inside the cells. As it is one of the antioxidants that cross into the brain, it can help protect the brain from oxidative damage and neuro-degenerative diseases. It may also help with the tissue injury that results from strokes. Lipoic acid has been shown to reduce cataract formation in some experimental models.

How to Take Lipoic Acid Typical doses of lipoic acid range from 300 to 1,000 mg per day. Doses of 1,000 mg are effective for diabetic peripheral neuropathy, and up to 1,200 mg per day have been effective in cardiac neuropathy. For some patients, 600 mg might be adequate. You will find capsules of many different sizes. I usually recommend taking 333-mg capsules, from one to three times a day, although it is not necessary to divide the dose. I often recommend that diabetics take lipoic acid with chromium and gamma-linolenic acid as well as other nutrients.

Melatonin

Melatonin is a hormone that is manufactured in the pineal gland from the amino acid tryptophan. The pineal gland is a pea-sized organ that sits at the base of the brain. Melatonin is also available as a dietary supplement. It is the substance that appears to regulate the "body clock," the physiological rhythm that relates to day/night changes.

Melatonin levels normally go up when it turns dark, and they are low during daylight hours. This hormone is also an antioxidant/free-radical scavenger that appears to slow the aging process. The production of melatonin is high in youth and declines steadily with age. Many signs of aging are associated with this loss of melatonin production, but cause and effect have not been proven. Large doses of melatonin have been administered to animals and humans without any known side effects.

Supplements of melatonin, taken at night, often help with insomnia and in overcoming symptoms of jet lag (for jet lag, it is taken near the bedtime in the new time zone for two or three days before departure and after arrival). Unlike most medications for insomnia, melatonin is not addictive. When it is used for insomnia, it does not leave you with any hangover or withdrawal symptoms, although a small percentage of people will report feeling sluggish the next morning or occasionally a paradoxical effect of worsened insomnia. Some animal and human studies have shown benefits in reducing cancer metastases and enhancing immune function. In animal studies, there is a clear increase in longevity (unfortunately, it is difficult to do longevity studies in humans). In humans, it has helped in treating depression, especially that associated with little exposure to light in the winter (seasonal affective disorder). It may help to lower eye pressures in patients with glaucoma.

How to Take Melatonin Melatonin is commonly available in 3-mg capsules or tablets, often in sublingual (under-the-tongue) form to dissolve in the mouth or in timed-release tablets. The usual melatonin dose is 3 mg at bedtime, but individual responses may be better with doses ranging from 1 to 6 mg. For insomnia or depression, if the dose you try does not work, you may need to increase or decrease the dose.

Some people seem to benefit from taking 10 to 15 mg of melatonin, without developing any apparent side effects. Larger doses are being studied for birth control because of melatonin's effect on sexual hormone balance.

Supplements of melatonin are almost all synthetically produced, but the synthetic molecules are identical to the natural human melatonin. There may be some brands on the market that contain actual animal pineal gland, but I do not recommend these as they are not as well standardized and may contain impurities. Synthetic melatonin supplements are pure white.

Methylsulfonyl-methane (MSM)

Methylsulfonyl-methane (MSM) is a source of sulfur, an essential nutrient. Sulfur is an essential component of connective tissue, antibodies, hair, nails, and many proteins. It is also part of many detoxifying pathways for environmental chemicals and drugs, and in the breakdown of used hormones. Although most people do not have any deficiency of sulfur, supplements may have therapeutic properties.

MSM is a derivative of DMSO, another sulfur compound that is commonly used as a solvent but also has antioxidant and anti-inflammatory properties. It produces a very strong sulfur or garlic smell in the sweat and breath that limits its usefulness. MSM has similar therapeutic properties without the associated smell.

MSM is commonly used for both osteoarthritis and rheumatoid arthritis, and other inflammatory processes such as lupus (SLE). It shows promise in the management of allergies, asthma, and diabetes, and many people find that it relieves their fibromyalgia symptoms. MSM inhibits the cross linking of collagen, a process that occurs with aging, and thus can prevent hardening of the connective tissue. As a result of this and its antioxidant properties, it may reduce the signs of aging in the skin.

How to Take MSM MSM is available in capsules of 500 mg and in pure powder. Typical doses range from 500 to 1,000 mg daily as a maintenance or preventive level, and up to 5,000 mg daily as a treatment for allergies, arthritis, and fibromyalgia syndrome. After a few days or weeks, the dose is reduced to maintenance levels. Some people find that they control their symptoms better if they continue to take MSM at 2,000 to 4,000 mg daily. A teaspoon of the pure powder contains just under 4,000 mg.

Phosphatidylserine (PS)

This is a phospholipid that is manufactured in the brain if the required components, such as B vitamins and fatty acids, are available in adequate quantities. It is important for maintaining healthy brain cell membranes and neurotransmitter activity. Supplements of PS are helpful with disorders of brain function, particularly in preserving memory in the elderly, such as in Alzheimer's disease, and in improving mood in depressed elderly patients.

How to Take Phosphatidylserine The typical dose of PS is 100 mg, two to three times a day for memory impairment and depression. Patients may see similar benefits with supplements of vitamin E and *Ginkgo biloba.* However, some patients have had significant improvement with phosphatidylserine in addition to these other nutrients. I often combine PS with *Ginkgo biloba* (see chapter 8) as part of a comprehensive health program for elderly patients.

Transfer Factor

Transfer factor is a collection of small proteinlike molecules found in white blood cells and in colostrum (the thick secretions that are part of the first breast milk for newborns) that act as immune messengers. They are called transfer factor because they "transfer" immune activity and infection resistance to the newborn so they have some protection before they have had time to develop their own immune system. Not only does transfer factor support the normal white blood cell function, it also increases interferon production. Interferon is the antiviral substance produced in response to viral infections.

These substances are found in all mammals, and they are not specific to the particular species, meaning that transfer factor from cows will be active in humans. Much of the research on transfer factor is done with that derived from white blood cells, called DLE (dialyzable leukocyte extract), and some is done on extracts from colostrum or colostrum itself. The transfer of immunity is based in part on the enhancement of immune cells and the "education" of the immune cells to be ready to fight back against infectious agents.

Transfer factor supplements are beneficial for any immune system disorders, including immune deficiency diseases such as HIV. It is also valuable for viral infections including Epstein-Barr virus (EBV), cytomegalovirus (CMV), other Herpes viruses, and upper respiratory viruses (colds and flu), as well as autoimmune or inflammatory diseases, such as lupus (SLE), bronchitis, asthma, and prostatitis.

Transfer factor is beneficial for chronic fatigue–immune deficiency syndrome (CFS or CFIDS), perhaps because it helps the immune dysregulation that goes along with the illness. Many patients with cancer do far better with high-dose supplements of transfer factor. Although the reports are mixed, transfer factor improves survival statistics for patients with a variety of tumors, even those that are already metastatic.

How To Take Transfer Factor Transfer factor is available in 200-mg capsules, and the typical dose for most patients is one to two capsules three times a day. For chronic fatigue patients these doses have been very helpful.

For cancer patients I have recommended nine capsules a day or more, but it is only part of a comprehensive approach to the treatment of cancer. HIV patients should be taking the higher levels similar to cancer patients. For an acute viral infection, you can increase the basic dose to six capsules per day.

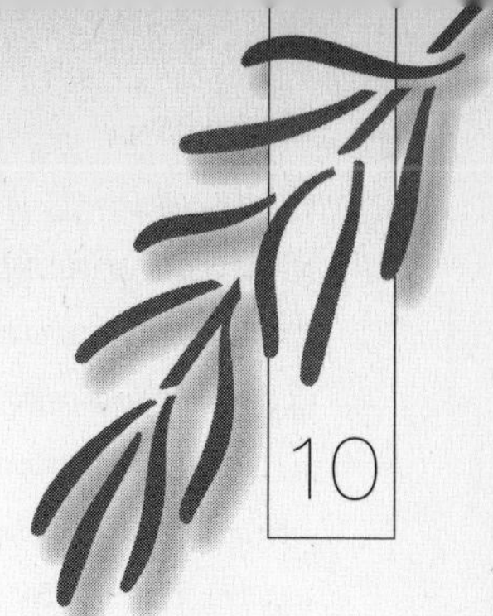

10

Practical Guidelines: Buying and Taking Supplements

When I recommend supplements, I often hear questions about where to get them and what brands to buy. How do you avoid being misled by unscrupulous manufacturers or overzealous sales pitches? Antagonists to dietary supplements sometimes leave you with the false impression that all manufacturers are disreputable. Nothing could be farther from the truth. In my experience, most supplement manufacturers are reliable and honest, and *they depend on good results from their products to generate repeat sales.* This does not mean that all products on the market are reliable, or that you won't find some exaggerated claims or some that are completely unfounded.

Manufacturers and Retailers

Most manufacturers of brand-name products in health food stores follow Good Manufacturing Practices (GMPs), and you should make sure they do before purchasing their products. The purpose of GMPs is to assure that what is on the label is in the product; that the product disintegrates and is bioavailable and unadulterated. Ask your retailer to find out from their manufacturers or suppliers. You can usually find reliable retail products at health food stores, through mail-order channels, and in professional offices. (Check Appendix 2 for sources.)

I have a lot of experience with supplements sold through professional offices. They are usually of high quality and are designed by the practitioners for their own method of practice. Practitioners sometimes have their own brand label, but most of the products will be similar to those of other practitioners and comparable to retail products. It is true that practitioners sometimes will charge higher prices for their products than retail store prices, assuming that they are more convenient for their clients, but they should not be markedly different from the products you can buy through other channels. Sometimes professional products are less expensive than those from other sources, but you should always compare doses to make sure you are getting the same quantity of the ingredients.

There are also good name brands available at health food stores, and some of the larger stores have their own in-house brand labels. Several mail-order sources supply brand names similar to the ones in health food stores, and some of the larger mail-order companies also have their own labels. Like the manufacturers, they also are dependent on good results to generate repeat business. The mail order companies usually discount from the full retail price, but local stores also frequently offer discounts. What you need to know is that *virtually all the raw materials for dietary supplements are made in bulk by a few manufacturers.* They are then purchased by supplement "manufacturers" who only tablet, encapsulate, and affix their own label to the products before sending them to distributors or retail outlets.

There was a time when there were more unscrupulous companies selling dietary supplements, but as the industry has matured they have formed trade groups to help monitor each other. Also, the consumer is becoming more sophisticated at evaluating supplements because there are frequent articles in newspapers and magazines on the topic, and a variety of excellent books for the consumer. Companies now have to keep on their toes if they are to stay in business, and they have to sell effective, competitive products. Dietary supplements are increasingly popular, and this has driven the market to provide more reliable products.

Be Wary of Claims

What this means most of the time is that the hyperbolic claims for particular brands are exaggerated, even though the ingredients are what they claim to be and do what they are supposed to. Some companies claim that their brand of "vitamin Z" is superior because of the form, or because it is "all natural," or it is combined with "synergistic nutrients" or herbs. Most of the time the additional dietary factors that are present are there in such small quantities that they have only a token presence—not enough to be therapeutic. If they are valuable in themselves, make sure the amount in the supplement is adequate to justify the price.

Some companies will say that their product is highly researched and tested (to justify a higher price), but when you look at the research papers that they provide, the studies refer to the basic nutrient ingredient (such as folic acid or beta-carotene) not to their particular brand. In these cases, I agree that their supplement is probably healthy and of great benefit, but so are many others on the market that are just as good and usually much less expensive.

What to Look for in Pricing

There have been in the past, and may still be, some very cheap mail-order supplements that did not meet the potency claims made on the label. This is much less likely now as the dietary supplement market has matured, but it is still possible. If a price looks too good to be true, it probably is. For example, if you price several reliable brands at between $9 and $12 per hundred capsules, and you find the same ingredients for $4 to $6 per hundred, you need to be very suspicious. On the other hand, if you find the same product for $19, you should also be aware that you may be paying too much. Sometimes a retailer will have special sales that make the price temporarily well below average. If the brand is reliable, take advantage of the sale, but continue to check the comparable price the next time you purchase, in case it has increased.

Most dietary supplement suppliers are very competitive, and a below-cost item may not meet label claim or on occasion may be made with inferior raw ingredients. These may have contamination problems or problems with disintegration and solubility. Synthetic vitamin E, for example, is much cheaper than the natural form, but the molecule is slightly different, and contains only the alpha-tocopherol, not the beta, gamma, or delta forms found in "mixed, natural tocopherols." That information should be on the label. The most likely supplements to be a problem are the most expensive ones, such as coenzyme Q_{10} or proanthocyanidins, or nonstandardized herbs which are generally much less expensive than the standardized products.

My advice is to seek a reliable mail-order company, a health food store, or a professional line of products from your practitioner, and check that the manufacturer follows GMPs in manufacturing. You can ask the sellers, who should be able to find out from the companies, if they do not already know. Also, make sure that they are hypoallergenic and that there are no extraneous ingredients such as artificial flavors, colors, sweeteners, or preservatives in the products. Although some of these may be safe, some of them are not, and their presence is a sign that the manufacturers are not as concerned with quality.

The Price of Health

I realize that supplement programs, even if you find them at the best prices, can be expensive by some standards. But I also know that people spend money on far less worthwhile items, often to the detriment of their health. I often suggest to my patients that they add up all that they spend on candy, sodas, doughnuts, coffee, cigarettes, alcohol, ice cream, cakes, cookies, and products of a similar nature.

I know that this total often adds up to quite a large expenditure spread out in little increments from day to day. (I know, because the average American consumes two doughnuts a day, one to two colas a day, more than one cup of coffee, plus twenty-three gallons of ice cream a year.) When they find out what they spend, frequently in the range of five to ten dollars a day, they learn that it would cover more than the cost of their entire health program, including office visits with me, supplements, and even organic foods. My conclusion is that supplements are an expense that can be completely covered by making healthier choices without any extra outlay of cash. I realize that for some people who do not make these poor choices, supplements may be a significant expenditure, and these comparisons are less meaningful to them, but the point is that affording supplements is usually a question of priorities.

Beyond these considerations, it is difficult to put a price on good health. Staying out of the doctor's office or out of the hospital is worth a lot of money, to say nothing of the anguish and discomfort that you want to avoid, and the more serious diseases that have graver consequences. So supplements may be seen as a great investment, and you may even save more than you spend on them by avoiding all that junk.

Timed-Release Supplements

Most "timed-release" products are not worth the extra money that you may spend on them. In fact, they may even be less effective than the plain variety. For example, in order to achieve the best effects with vitamin C, especially in viral infections, you sometimes need a very high blood level. These levels are more difficult to achieve with timed-release pills, because of their slow dissolution and absorption.

Occasionally timed-release pills are not properly timed, so that the tablet does not disintegrate and dissolve in time or in the right place to be well absorbed from the intestinal tract. Most plain supplements are fairly well absorbed and utilized, so a slow-release form is unnecessary. There are two exceptions to this that are worth mentioning. One is vitamin B_3, or niacin, which can cause a temporary flush of the skin, but is less likely to do so in timed-release form. (Remember, however, that the timed-release form is more likely to cause liver problems in some people.) The other valuable timed-release supplement is iron, which often causes some constipation and indigestion in plain form. It is usually better tolerated as timed-release iron carbonyl. The common drug-store variety, iron sulfate, seems to be the worst for causing constipation and is the least well absorbed.

Combination Supplements

Except for a multivitamin and a few simple combinations, it is better to take your individual nutrients in separate pills. This makes it easier to change the dose of one nutrient without having to alter many others at the same time. It is almost invariably less expensive to take separate nutrients, but you can expect to take from six to ten pills twice per day for a comprehensive, basic supplement program. This is assuming you are healthy. If you have a health problem, you might end up taking ten to fifteen pills twice a day. For vigorous longevity programs, you may end up taking quite a few more.

Manufacturers make specific combinations to distinguish their product from others—to establish a position, or "market niche." Such "exclusive" products can often command a higher price. Do not be drawn in by their exaggerated claims. A product may well have all the claimed benefits, but is it worth the price? Compare the ingredients (mg to mg, or IU to IU) and the price. Once you have an established program with which you are satisfied, then you might find a few combinations that meet your needs, and you can use them to reduce the number of pills that you take.

If you find that a particular brand works for you and it is reasonably priced, stay with it. You might want to ask your health practitioner for advice. If you haven't tried comparable products, you would be wise to shop around for price. Ask how long a brand has been on the market. Most of the reliable companies have been around for a while. (Of course, new reliable companies do appear in the marketplace.)

When to Take Supplements

Most of the time, it is a good idea to take supplements with food. Nutrients occur in nature as combinations with each other and with other substances in foods. Generally, they work together in digestion, absorption, and other physiological processes. Also, it is much easier on the digestion process to take supplements with food. Supplements are concentrated, and sometimes they can cause digestive upset or abdominal discomfort when taken in large doses on an empty stomach.

Single nutrients, such as vitamin C, can usually be taken at any time, in almost any dose, without upsetting your system. Taking a drink of pure vitamin C powder mixed with diluted fruit juice is actually refreshing, and it is an easy way to take a large dose.

Sometimes, there is antagonism or competition for absorption between different nutrients, such as copper and zinc, or in utilization, for example, iron and vitamin E. However, these are usually not sufficient to be a serious concern when taking large doses of supplements.

There are some exceptions to this rule. For example, some of the amino acids are better utilized for specific purposes when taken separately from foods. (See chapter 7.) My recommendation is not to worry too much about such combinations; they are generally minor, and worrying about them makes supplement programs confusing and inconvenient. If you do not remember to take things, they are not going to do you any good.

You may have concerns about swallowing so many pills if you are on many different supplements. If you have difficulty, it is easiest to take them with a thicker liquid, such as tomato juice or a blended fruit and yogurt smoothee. This usually makes it easy to open the throat for swallowing and it coats the pills, making it easier for them to go down. After you are able to take them this way, it becomes easy to swallow many pills at one time, even with plain water, but be careful. (One of my patients uses this trick—just before taking the liquid for the pills she says to herself, "I am really thirsty." She says it helps the pills go down.)

Supplements During Pregnancy

Most pregnant women need extra nutrition, and most physicians will recommend at least some dietary supplements. As stated before, folic acid is essential for the prevention of some birth defects, and other nutrients are helpful in preventing pre-eclampsia (toxemia of pregnancy; see the discussion of B_6 and magnesium). Some supplements are helpful in reducing morning sickness, especially pyridoxine (vitamin B_6) and ginger.

Most of the nutrients on basic supplement programs are helpful during pregnancy and are often recommended by obstetricians. Extra iron and calcium are useful additions to a routine supplement program. Although commonly prescribed prenatal vitamins contain the conventionally recommended amounts of nutrients, they are relatively low compared to the amounts found in a basic multiple. The only precaution is to avoid taking too much vitamin A during the first three months of pregnancy. Anything above 10,000 IU may be too much, but this only applies to preformed vitamin A, not to beta-carotene. Many herbs are considered more risky in pregnancy because they have not been formally studied. Most of the common ones are probably very safe, but there is not enough information to make a specific recommendation at this time.

How to Store Supplements

You do not need to take special precautions when storing most dietary supplements. It is usually sufficient to keep them on a shelf in a pantry or on the kitchen counter. Most of the products are quite stable if kept in dry, room-temperature conditions, out of direct sunlight. Most supplement bottles are opaque, providing protection from light, but direct sunlight even through a window will heat the contents of the bottle. As with any food, do not leave them for prolonged periods in a hot car or in a closed carrier out in the sun, where they will also easily get overheated.

Sometimes people are tempted to put their supplements in the refrigerator, but this is not a good idea. Every time you open a bottle of cold supplement pills in a warm external environment, there will be some condensation on the surface of the pills that remain in the bottle. Eventually, they will become wet and sticky, or they will actually begin to dissolve, depending on how much they attract moisture. An exception is some supplements of intestinal flora (lactobacilli or bifidobacteria) that sometimes keep better in the cold.

For the same reason, do not keep your supplements in the bathroom (not that you were really tempted to do so). It gets too humid with all the showering to keep them dry and fresh. The best place for storage is probably the kitchen, since it is usually dry, and it is convenient, since you will take most of your supplements with meals.

How Long Do Supplements Keep?

It is not a good idea to keep supplements for a long time after they have been opened. Although some are quite stable in a dry environment, there is inevitably some oxidation and loss of potency. The amount of loss depends on the particular nutrient. Many of the supplements are quite stable, and last for years if kept cool and dry. Minerals do not deteriorate with time.

With some products, the surface of the pill will change color when some components oxidize. When this happens, the surface of the tablets usually becomes darker and mottled. You should discard these tablets. You can also see this kind of discoloration inside of some two-part capsules, and you should discard these also. (Some products normally have a mixed-color surface, and you should get to know what they look like when you first buy them so you will know when they change.)

The best course of action is to buy what you need for a one- to three-month period or up to six or eight months if it is more convenient, and store unopened bottles in a cool (but not necessarily refrigerated), dark room. If you buy a large amount, you may keep the unopened bottles in the refrigerator, but be sure to bring them to room temperature before opening them, and don't store them in the fridge once they have been opened.

Multicompartment Storage Boxes

One last note that will make it easier for you to take supplements if you are taking more than a few: There are multi-compartment storage containers, similar to fishing tackle or sewing boxes, but with a rubber gasket seal to keep out air. They come with six to sixteen chambers to hold a number of different supplements. Label each chamber unless you clearly recognize the different supplements. If you have too many for the box, you can mix two in one chamber as long as you recognize the difference.

The advantage of having one of these multicompartment boxes is that you only have to open one lid each time you want to take your supplements. Since you might be taking many different products at one time, this is an enormous time saver. And if you have arthritis, it will help reduce the stress on your hands from opening so many bottles so frequently (of course, some of the supplements will help with the arthritis).

Another way to accomplish this is to purchase some empty pharmacy vials and set aside some time to fill up a one-week supply of morning and evening doses all at once. It is a good idea to have different-size vials for your morning and evening for recognition, in case the doses are different. You can also use small zip-lock jeweler's bags for daily doses.

Both of these methods have one further advantage in that the original storage bottle for each supplement is opened less frequently, reducing exposure of the main supply to air and humidity. You should not have great difficulty keeping supplements safely.

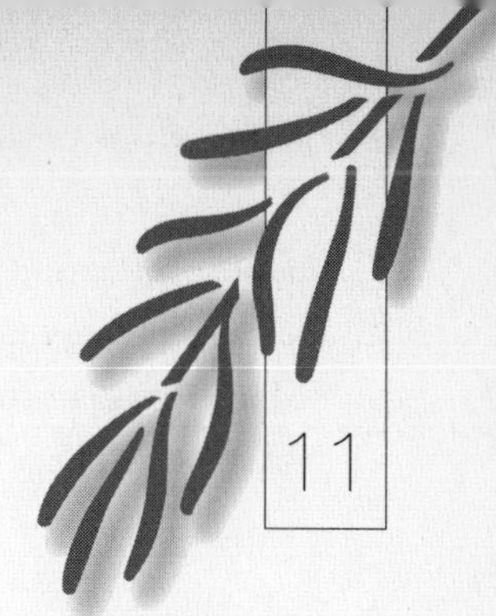

11

Your Personal Supplement Program

WITH ALL THIS INFORMATION, how do you go about setting up a personal dietary supplement program for yourself? There are so many different supplements and so many approaches to health programs that it may seem confusing. Many sources of information on supplements will tell you of the value of some of them, but will leave you unsure of where to begin your own program. Because of this confusion, many people give up in frustration, but *it is important to your health to get started now.*

In this chapter you will find some basic guidelines and some sample programs for health enhancement and preventive medicine. You will also find some sample treatment programs for specific conditions. Consider them as guidelines, not prescriptions. When reading these recommendations, always keep in mind that your particular needs may require more or less than what you see here. This is for both the specific supplements you might need and the amounts of any one of them.

If you are a physician, remember: *It is an error to try to treat diagnoses rather than people.* Everyone is an individual, and frequently health problems occur in combinations. There are also specific life situations that demand personal attention in designing a health program. Keep this in mind when recommending supplements or any other health program for your patients. More physician training is available in this field, especially through the American College for Advancement in Medicine. (See Appendix 2.)

Supplements Are Supplements

First, a reminder that supplements are just that: additions to a healthy diet and support for many health practices. They neither replace good foods nor eliminate the need for exercise, stress management, laughter, and a positive attitude. I have often known people who think that supplements could relieve them of the discipline required to change their health habits. No single health practice cures or prevents all illness and degeneration, even though any one of them will help to some degree.

Second, remember to *keep any health program simple* enough to follow. If you make it too complex, chances are you will fall off the program and lose all the potential benefits. Take any dietary supplements at breakfast, dinner, or bedtime, unless you have unusual discipline and can remember lunchtime doses. There is some small benefit in absorption of nutrients from dividing your intake of water-soluble supplements into three daily doses, but *not* if you do not remember to take them.

If you do not eat breakfast, it is time to reconsider your health habits, since breakfast is an important meal. Even if it is just a piece of fruit with some whole-grain toast and a few almonds, or some whole-grain cereal, try to eat something to start your day. If you absolutely cannot face food before noon, take the first dose of supplements with your lunch and the second dose with your evening meal about six to eight hours later.

Program for General Prevention

For general preventive medicine, you may wish to start with the basic supplements essential for health promotion, assuming that you are in good health. These would be the Basic Multiple formula (see page 24 for a breakdown of the nutrients in the Basic Multiple), some extra vitamins C and E, and probably some natural carotenoids (if your multi differs from the

Basic Multiple, simply adjust doses of the different nutrients). The extra E and carotenoids can be taken any time of day, since they are fat soluble and not rapidly turned over. If you do not divide the water-soluble supplements into at least two doses per day, some of them will be less well absorbed and excreted more rapidly. They will still benefit you, but perhaps not as much. If you are concerned that you might not tolerate some of the supplements because of unusual sensitivities, you might wish to start with one at a time for a few days. If you wish, take one formula, as indicated below, for two or three days, and if there is no problem with that one add another for two or three days, and so on. The following table represents such a basic supplement program:

SUPPLEMENT	A.M.	P.M.
Basic Multiple Formula	3	3
Natural carotenoids 25,000 IU		1
Vitamin C 1,000 mg	2	2
Vitamin E 400 IU natural, mixed	1	

Program for Stronger Protection

If you wish to pursue a stronger preventive medicine program, if you exercise heavily, if you are exposed to toxic chemicals in your environment, or are under unusual emotional stress, it is advisable to take extra supplements. Vitamins E and C, an essential fatty acid supplement, and a few other antioxidants, such as the mixed bioflavonoids, are likely to be helpful. I would also recommend additional magnesium and some coenzyme Q_{10}, especially if you are over forty years old. This supplement program is represented in the following table.

SUPPLEMENT	A.M.	P.M.
Basic Multiple Formula	3	3
Bioflavonoid mix 1,000 mg	1	1
Coenzyme Q_{10} 50 to 100 mg		1
GLA 240 mg (borage oil)		1
Magnesium aspartate 200 mg		1

Natural carotenoids 25,000 IU		1
Vitamin C 1,000 mg	3	3
Vitamin E 400 IU natural, mixed	1	1

Program for Vigorous Life Enhancement

For more vigorous protection from free radicals and to slow or even reverse some of the effects of aging, you will need extra dietary supplements and higher doses of some. Include additional vitamin C and magnesium, higher amounts of coenzyme Q_{10}, and some more phytochemical flavonoids, as reflected in the following table:

SUPPLEMENT	A.M.	P.M.
Basic Multiple Formula	3	3
Bioflavonoid mix 1,000 mg	1	1
Coenzyme Q_{10} 100 to 200 mg		1
GLA 240 mg (borage oil)		1
Magnesium aspartate 200 mg	1	1
Natural carotenoids 25,000 IU	1	
Proanthocyanidins 50 mg mixed	1	1
Quercetin 400 mg		1
Siberian ginseng 200 mg Std.	1	1
Vitamin C 1,000 mg	4	4
Vitamin E 400 IU natural, mixed	1	1

As You Age

These previous programs are by no means the most extreme programs that some people are following. As you age, for example into your fifties and sixties, you may wish to add those nutrients that further help to protect memory, vision, liver function, and gastrointestinal health, in addition to preventing cancer, diabetes, heart disease, and stroke. This further list of supplements might include extra selenium, *Ginkgo biloba,* silymarin, bilberry, glutamine, melatonin, and carnitine. Admittedly, this is a vigorous program with many pills to take and greater expense. However, even if it were ten or twelve dollars a day, it would still be less than what some people spend on cigarettes, coffee, colas, hotdogs, and doughnuts! The following table represents such a program:

SUPPLEMENT	A.M.	P.M.
Basic Multiple Formula	3	3
Bilberry 100 mg	1	1
Bioflavonoid mix 1,000 mg	1	1
Coenzyme Q_{10} *200 mg*		1
Ginkgo biloba *extract 60 mg*	1	1
GLA 240 mg (from borage oil)	1	
L-carnitine 500 mg	1	1
L-glutamine 500 mg	2	2
Magnesium aspartate 200 mg	1	1
Melatonin 3 mg		1 *or* 2
Natural carotenoids 25,000 IU	1	1
Proanthocyanidins 50 mg mixed	1	1
Quercetin 400 mg	1	1
Selenium 200 mcg		1
Siberian ginseng 200 mg Std.	1	1
Silymarin 150 mg (80 percent standardized)	1	1
Vitamin C 1,000 mg	4	4
Vitamin E 400 IU natural, mixed	1	1

If you have specific health problems, it is important to have them diagnosed first. If they are chronic degenerative conditions, or your health practitioner says, “Well, what do you expect at your age?” then it is time to consider some of the therapeutic supplements that are described in the previous chapters. (You might also try to find a more responsive health practitioner.)

Your attempt to enhance your health is not a substitute for diagnosis and proper treatment of medical conditions. You can, however, enhance your health and increase the likelihood of success of any other treatment regimen. You will also probably decrease the side effects of medication and increase the rate of healing after surgery or other treatment.

Treatment Programs

When patients come to me for advice about specific medical problems, they usually have been told that they need medication or surgery, and they are seeking ways to avoid those treatments. Sometimes they have already tried medications, which have produced significant side effects.

Usually, they have many treatment alternatives but they have no information about their choices. One example of effective alternatives is the reduction in blood pressure that meditation produces. Others are the dietary changes and exercise programs that lead to lowered cholesterol. Since the medical treatments for these two conditions are sometimes more dangerous than the problems, it is worth seeking safer alternatives.

Dr. Dean Ornish has shown that patients with heart disease can often avoid surgery and reverse their heart disease with a combination of a low-fat diet, meditation, and exercise. Norman Cousins healed his ankylosing spondylitis (a form of arthritis of the spine) with laughter and high doses of vitamin C. He wrote about his experience in an article for the *New England Journal of Medicine,* and followed this article with a book, *The Anatomy of an Illness.* Many patients have cured their digestive disturbances simply by avoiding certain foods.

Over and over, we are seeing the results of lifestyle changes in health care. A recent scientific medical conference put on by the American College for Advancement in Medicine was titled: Lifestyle Medicine—Medicine for the Nineties. Researchers and physicians both attended and taught at this scientific meeting. Much of it related to the role of dietary supplements in medical therapy. Ongoing conferences at ACAM into the new millennium have further confirmed this trend, and major medical institutions are now adding lectures on supplements to their programs and establishing alternative-medicine divisions at hospitals and medical schools.

Dietary supplements are among the safest and most effective choices in health care. They are almost free of side effects, they are easy to take, they are relatively inexpensive, and they usually enhance many life functions besides the specific condition for which they are being given. Here are some examples of how nutritionally oriented physicians might use supplements as part of the treatment for some specific health problems. These are suggestions that are supported in the medical literature and by the experience of many physicians.

Remember that these are examples, not prescriptions for you, and the supplement list is in addition to many other health practices. Other supplements may be helpful, and you may not need all of these to get results. You might try some of the suggestions, and then add more or change to others on the lists if you are not improving as much as you expect. For more information on any one supplement, look for its description in previous chapters. No one program is appropriate for everybody, but these suggestions are good starting points from which individual programs can be modified.

Allergies and Asthma

Since allergies and asthma are so often related, and the therapeutic supplements are so similar, they are linked in the discussion. Allergic symptoms may be as simple as hay fever or sinus congestion. They may be precipitants of sinus infections. Asthmatic wheezing is more serious. Stress reduction frequently plays a large role in the management of asthma, and attacks may be precipitated by stress or a respiratory infection. Food allergies are also common complicating factors. In children, the most common foods that cause asthmatic responses are milk, eggs, peanuts, soy, and wheat. In adults, research does not show milk to be as common, but many patients report that milk or wheat causes symptoms.

Asthma may be severe, and it is unwise to stop your medication unless symptoms are well controlled. Supplement doses may need to be increased, such as extra quercetin or nettle, to manage allergic responses. You can take extra nettle as needed for symptoms as they occur. Occasionally, someone is sensitive to a specific supplement. This is unpredictable, so be on the lookout for reactions. The most valuable supplements, and their recommended doses, are charted below:

SUPPLEMENT	A.M.	P.M.
Basic Multiple Formula	3	3
Coenzyme Q_{10} 100 to 200 mg	1	

GLA 240 mg (from borage oil)	1	
Magnesium aspartate 200 mg	1	1
Nettle 250 mg (as needed)	2	2
Proanthocyanidins 50 mg mixed	1	1
Pyridoxine (B_6) 250 mg	1	
Quercetin 400 mg	1	1
Transfer factor 200 mg	1	1
Vitamin C 1,000 mg	3	3
Vitamin E 400 IU natural mixed	1	1

Angina/Hardening of the Arteries

Arteriosclerotic heart disease and other vascular diseases result from the buildup of plaque (fatty, fibrous, and calcified tissue) in the coronary arteries and the arteries to the brain, abdomen, pelvic organs, and legs. As mentioned earlier, it may be caused or reversed by many lifestyle habits. Common symptoms of heart disease include chest tightness or pain, which may radiate to the left arm, jaw, or chin; shortness of breath; and fatigue. Sometimes the symptom is described as a pressure sensation, or even as heartburn or indigestion. These symptoms are usually precipitated by exertion, stress, or even a large meal.

Cerebral artery disease leads to faintness, loss of mental function, a brief loss of brain function called a transient ischemic attack (TIA), and strokes. Hardening of the arteries to the pelvic organs can lead to sexual dysfunction, and leg arterial disease leads to pain in the calves when walking and poor circulation to the feet, which may end up as gangrene. Chelation therapy with intravenous EDTA can make a great difference for patients who have hardening of the arteries. Doctors who do chelation therapy can be found through the American College for Advancement in Medicine (see Resources). They can also provide more information on this treatment. It is always used in conjunction with lifestyle changes and supplements.

It is essential to have good cardiology and vascular evaluations in addition to any health enhancement program. Depending on the symptoms and history, the supplement program may be quite variable, but the following list includes those supplements that are most likely to be beneficial:

SUPPLEMENT	A.M.	P.M.
Basic Multiple Formula	3	3
Arginine 500 mg	2–4	2–4
Coenzyme Q_{10} 200 mg	1	
Ginkgo biloba *extract 60 mg*	1	1
GLA 240 mg (from borage oil)	1	
Hawthorn berry 250 mg	1	1
L-carnitine 250 mg	2	2
Magnesium aspartate 200 mg	1	1
Natural carotenoids 25,000 IU	1	
Niacin-inositol 400 mg	2	2
Proanthocyanidins 50 mg mixed	1	1
Taurine 500 mg	2	2
Vitamin C 1,000 mg	3	3
Vitamin E 400 IU natural, mixed	1	1

Anxiety/Depression

There are many different reasons that someone might be anxious or depressed, and this is not meant to be a prescription for all forms of either. Anxiety and depression often go together, but not always. Physiological problems that might lead to anxiety and depression include food or environmental allergies, hypoglycemia, candidiasis, chemical or heavy metal toxicity, hypo- or hyperthyroidism, inadequate sleep, and many illnesses. Listlessness, fatigue, appetite and sleep disturbances, low motivation, and loss of libido characterize depression. In its most serious form it may lead to suicidal thoughts. Mental health professionals can be a great help in getting through the emotional components of anxiety and depression.

Frequently, simple improvement in your general health status through diet, exercise, and relaxation techniques makes a great difference in depression and anxiety. Follow a healthy, whole foods diet and avoid alcohol and caffeine. Supplements of vitamin C, B-complex, essential fatty acids, and many other nutrients can help, and many herbs also help with mood problems. In the elderly, extra vitamin B_{12} frequently helps with depression and fatigue. Serious psychiatric depression may require medication, but many nutrients and botanical products can also provide relief and in some circumstances can substitute for the medications.

The following table lists supplements that often help with anxiety or mild to moderate depression. Higher doses of some supplements may help with the more severe conditions. You may need less than the doses listed, and in some cases more. Start with a lower dose and increase if necessary. I suggest trying either St. John's wort or 5-HTP for depression, not both, and kava if anxiety is your major symptom. You may have to vary the combinations for your individual needs, as this can be a complex problem. In addition to the basic health program, consider taking the following supplements:

SUPPLEMENT	A.M.	P.M.
5-HTP 50 mg	1 *or* 2	1 *or* 2
Kava 250 mg	1	1 *or* 2
Magnesium aspartate 200 mg	1	1
Niacinamide 500 mg	1	1
St. John's wort 300 mg	1	2

Arthritis

Inflammation or deterioration of the joints, with progressive destruction of the joint cartilage, is responsible for much of the disability of the elderly, although it also affects younger people. As the cartilage gets worn away, the bones of the joints rub on each other and cause varying degrees of pain.

Rheumatoid arthritis is the result of connective tissue destruction by immune complexes formed when the immune system attacks the body's own tissue. This is called autoimmunity, which is poor regulation (or *dysregulation*) of immune function, not simply increased activity. Some dietary supplements that enhance immune activity actually relieve rheumatoid arthritis and reduce joint destruction, since they help restore normal immune regulation.

Rheumatoid arthritis is more common in women than men, and occurs in relatively young people, most commonly starting in the thirties and forties. It is commonly associated with other immune system disorders, such as dry-eye syndrome (Sjögren's syndrome) and Raynaud's phenomenon (spasms in the blood vessels of the hands or feet, usually brought on by exposure to cold).

Food allergies commonly play a role in causing rheumatoid arthritis. Although many physicians and the well-known national arthritis organizations often say that diet has nothing to do with arthritis, clinical experience and a number of research articles have shown otherwise. Healthy diets and avoiding food allergens are important components of arthritis treatment. Allergy tests can help pinpoint which foods to avoid. In my experience, dairy products and meats make symptoms worse, possibly because of allergy and possibly because land-animal fats can increase inflammation.

Other immune arthritis conditions include ankylosing spondylitis (arthritis of the spine) and arthritis associated with psoriasis. Osteoarthritis, or degenerative joint disease, is more common than rheumatoid arthritis and is the result of wear and tear, infection, or joint injury. After the age of seventy, there is X-ray evidence of osteoarthritis in 85 percent of Americans, although some of them may have no symptoms. It is often helped by the same dietary supplements that relieve rheumatoid arthritis.

MSM had been reported to help with arthritis, and I have seen some patients benefit from 1,000 to 2,000 mg daily, after a few weeks of a higher dose, such as 4,000 mg twice a day. It is not clear whether it makes a difference when someone is already taking glucosamine sulfate and the other nutrients.

Many personal reports suggest other supplements that sometimes help arthritis. They include alfalfa tablets, extracts of sea cucumber, green-lipped mussel, and cartilage—from either shark or calf (bovine) sources. Some of my patients have reported benefits from these supplements. You can try these in addition to or instead of the program outlined below. The following supplements are often helpful for relieving symptoms and restoring joint integrity:

SUPPLEMENT	A.M.	P.M.
Basic Multiple Formula	3	3
EPA fish oil 1,000 mg	2	2
GLA 240 mg (from borage oil)	1	
Glucosamine sulfate 500 mg	2	2

Magnesium aspartate 200 mg	1	1
Niacinamide 500 mg	2	2
Proanthocyanidins 50 mg mixed	1	1
Vitamin C 1,000 mg	3	3
Vitamin E 400 IU natural mixed	1	1

CANDIDIASIS (YEAST OVERGROWTH)

The overgrowth of yeast in the intestinal tract (as mentioned in the section on grapefruit seed extract) can lead to a variety of symptoms as a result of the toxins that yeasts produce (mycotoxins). These symptoms are the result of allergy or toxins, not yeast in the bloodstream or organs. It is sometimes difficult to reduce the intestinal yeast population, but there are several dietary supplements that can help.

In addition to the supplements, it is important to reduce dietary and medical sources of yeast growth stimulants, such as antibiotics, hormones, and a high intake of sugar. Hormones or antibiotics may be necessary for medical reasons, but the resulting yeast overgrowth needs to be controlled. Of course, refined, white sugar is always avoidable, with a little determination, if you really want to keep it out of your diet.

Although they may be combined with medications when indicated, the following supplements are commonly used to help control the yeast overgrowth:

SUPPLEMENT	A.M.	P.M.
Grapefruit seed extract 100 mg	2	2
Lactobacillus acidophilus *(4 billion organisms per capsule)*	2	2
Garlic (deodorized) 500 mg	2	2
GLA 240 mg (as borage oil)	1	1

I often recommend a mixture of *Lactobacillus acidophilus* with the *Bifidobacterium bifidum*, either in capsule or powder form. This combination helps both the large and small intestines. The dose of powder is usually ½ teaspoon twice per day at the start of treatment and ⅓ teaspoon twice per day after some improvement. In addition to these specifics, I would recommend that you take the usual general health supplements and immune-enhancing supplements such as the following:

SUPPLEMENT	A.M.	P.M.
Basic Multiple Formula	3	3
Echinacea 250 mg	2	2
Magnesium aspartate 200 mg	1	1
Pyridoxine (B_6) 250 mg	1	
Vitamin C 1,000 mg	3	3
Vitamin E 400 IU	1	

These supplements and several others may be indicated for the management of various symptoms that people with candidiasis often experience. It is important to have a proper diagnosis, in case your symptoms are from other causes.

CONGESTIVE HEART FAILURE

The inability of the heart muscle to pump out all the blood that is returned through the veins is called congestive heart failure. Fluid is forced out of the blood vessels into the surrounding tissues by the buildup of pressure. The symptoms are shortness of breath, fatigue, swelling of the ankles, distended veins, difficulty breathing while lying down, and coughing.

Swelling of the legs occurs when the smaller right chamber (ventricle) of the heart is involved, because of the backup of blood coming into the heart from the legs, but both the right and left ventricles may be involved at the same time. Prevention is based on a healthy diet and maintaining both a good exercise program and normal weight, although some congenital abnormalities of the heart or damaged heart valves may also lead to heart failure.

For treatment, it is important to avoid salt in the diet to reduce excess fluid accumulation. There are several dietary supplements that can help treat heart failure, but it is important to have a proper diagnosis and medical management, since this can be a serious situation. Helpful supplements for treatment include:

SUPPLEMENT	A.M.	P.M.
Basic Multiple Formula	3	3
L-arginine 500 mg capsules	2	2
Coenzyme Q_{10} 200 mg	1	
Hawthorn berry 250 mg	2	1
Magnesium aspartate 200 mg	1	1
Taurine 500 mg	3	3
Vitamin C 1,000 mg	3	3
Vitamin E 400 IU natural, mixed	1	1

Higher doses of coenzyme Q_{10} or L-arginine may be important with more advanced heart failure. Again, other supplements are helpful with conditions that either cause or accompany heart failure, and they should be considered based on individual needs.

Diabetes

Diabetes mellitus (sometimes called "sugar diabetes") is a failure to properly metabolize sugar, specifically blood glucose. It results from either the reduced function of the pancreas, which produces insulin, or more commonly from inability of the cells to respond to insulin, called *insulin resistance.* Insulin is essential to move sugar out of the bloodstream into the muscles, where it can be burned for energy.

There are many causes of diabetes, the most common form of which is adult onset, which is almost always the result of poor health habits and being overweight. The symptoms of diabetes are excessive thirst and hunger, and frequent urination. Most of the time, adult-onset diabetes does not require insulin or the oral medications that are used to control blood sugar, and most people can be taken off medication if they follow the right diet (high fiber, high complex carbohydrate, low fat) and if they exercise.

In addition to lifestyle changes, there are specific supplements that help diabetics to control their blood sugar and to prevent the later complications, such as eye and vascular disorders, and diabetic neuropathy—a degeneration of the nerves leading to numbness and tingling starting in the feet and legs. Even Type I diabetics (juvenile type, or insulin dependent) can reduce their insulin doses with a complete approach to blood sugar management. Nonetheless, medical supervision of diabetes is usually essential, and I do not recommend trying to manage diabetes yourself. Tell your doctor what supplements you are taking. You don't need to ask permission, but your doctor should know if there are any potential interactions with medications, or if you can even lower the dose of some of them as a result of the supplements. If your doctor is nutritionally oriented, you may well receive some further advice on your supplement program. The following supplements may contribute to sugar control and prevention or management of diabetic complications:

SUPPLEMENT	A.M.	P.M.
Basic Multiple Formula	3	3
Bilberry 100 mg	1	1
Bioflavonoid mix 1,000 mg	1	1
Chromium 200 mcg	2	2
Coenzyme Q_{10} *200 mg*	1	
Ginkgo biloba *extract 60 mg*	1	1
GLA 240 mg (from borage oil)	1	
Lipoic acid 333 mg	1	2
Magnesium aspartate 200 mg	1	1
Proanthocyanidins 50 mg mixed	1	1
Quercetin 400 mg	1	1
Silymarin 150 mg (80% standardized)	1	1
Vitamin C 1,000 mg	3	3
Vitamin E 400 IU natural, mixed	1	1

DIGESTIVE DISORDERS

There are many varieties of digestive problems, including inflammatory diseases (Crohn's disease, ulcerative colitis, diverticulitis), acid indigestion (heartburn), peptic ulcers, hiatal hernia, irritable colon, lactose intolerance, yeast overgrowth, food allergies, and others. No one program is suitable for all these digestive problems.

Some of the most commonly prescribed drugs are those that are supposed to help with acid indigestion and ulcers, but these medications are overused and often improperly prescribed. Aspirin and nonsteroidal anti-inflammatory drugs are common causes of serious gastrointestinal bleeding. There are many nondrug treatments that help with a variety of gastrointestinal disorders. Some of the generally helpful dietary supplements are listed in the following table:

SUPPLEMENT	A.M.	P.M.
Basic Multiple Formula	3	3
Deglycyrrhizinated licorice 1 to 2 tabs for heartburn	*chew as needed*	
Garlic deodorized 500 mg	2	2
GLA 240 mg (as borage oil)	1	
Lactobacillus (4 billion organisms per capsule)	2	2
L-glutamine 500 mg	3	3
Magnesium aspartate 200 mg	1	1
Pyridoxine (B_6) 250 mg	1	
Vitamin C 1,000 mg	3	3
Vitamin E 400 IU natural, mixed	1	1

Fatigue

One of the most common complaints in any medical practice is fatigue (usually for both the patient and the doctor). There are many causes of persistent fatigue, as opposed to simply being tired from exercise or a heavy workload. There may be a serious medical disorder such as anemia, diabetes, heart disease, cancer, chronic fatigue/immune-dysfunction syndrome (also called CFIDS), hypothyroidism, and infection.

Some chronic everyday problems may also cause significant ongoing fatigue, such as stress, dietary imbalance, food allergy, nutritional deficiency, environmental toxicity, low blood sugar (hypoglycemia), and low-grade depression. Sometimes the problem is as simple as a lack of adequate exercise or boredom.

There are some general principles for reducing fatigue after eliminating any of the serious medical conditions as the underlying cause. Again, eating properly, exercising, and reducing emotional stressors can help increase your energy. Avoiding food allergens and environmental toxins helps reduce exposure to the chemical stressors. A general dietary supplement is often adequate to help reduce fatigue due to nutritional imbalances or borderline deficiencies.

Do not ignore the need to find out if persistent fatigue is the result of a serious medical problem. Treatment may require medical management in addition to lifestyle change and dietary supplements. The following supplement program often helps with fatigue from many causes, including chronic fatigue syndrome:

SUPPLEMENT	A.M.	P.M.
Basic Multiple Formula	3	3
Chromium 200 mcg	1	1
Coenzyme Q_{10} 100 mg	1	
GLA 240 mg (from borage oil)	1	
L-carnitine 250 mg	2	2
L-glutamine 500 mg	2	2
Magnesium aspartate 200 mg	1	1
Niacin, timed release, 250 mg	1	1
St. John's wort 300 mg	1	2
Transfer factor 200 mg	2	2
Vitamin C 1,000 mg	2	2
Vitamin E 400 IU natural, mixed	1	1

HEADACHES

As with fatigue, there are many causes of headaches. The most common problems are tension- or stress-related headaches and migraine headaches. Assuming there are no brain tumors, hypertension, or infections, such as meningitis, which can cause acute headaches, treatment with lifestyle changes and dietary supplements is often effective.

Migraines are called vascular headaches because they result from blood vessel spasms. There are many triggers that can precipitate migraine headaches. Common ones are caffeine, alcohol (especially red wine), chocolate, and sugar. Food allergies can also lead to a migraine, as can exposure to bright or flickering lights, lack of sleep, or emotional and psychological stress.

Most effective programs for headache control, other than drug treatments, rely on prevention. The pain-killer medications that are often used to treat migraines (Advil, Motrin, ibuprofen—all of which have the same active ingredient) have actually been shown to increase the severity and frequency of the headaches in people who use them often. This is possibly through some rebound effect that leads to even more use of the medications. The following supplement program is often effective for the drug-free management of migraines and may also help in the treatment of other headaches:

SUPPLEMENT	A.M.	P.M.
Basic Multiple Formula	3	3
Feverfew 250 mg standardized	1	1
Ginkgo biloba *extract 60 mg*	1	1
GLA 240 mg (from borage oil)	1	
Magnesium aspartate 200 mg	1	1
Niacin, timed release, 250 mg	1	1
Pyridoxine 250 mg	1	
Riboflavin 100 mg	2	2
Vitamin C 1,000 mg	2	2
Vitamin E 400 IU natural, mixed	1	

Hypertension (High Blood Pressure)

High blood pressure, even if mild, is associated with an increased risk of vascular diseases, including heart disease and stroke. The pressures are read as the *systolic,* which is the first number (when the heart pumps), and the *diastolic,* the second number (between beats). Disease risks are increased whenever the diastolic pressure is above 80. Such elevations are related to excess salt, sugar, caffeine, and animal fat in the diet, and obesity, which are all very common in the United States. They are also related to stress, smoking, alcohol consumption, and sedentary lifestyles.

Hypertension usually has no symptoms in early stages. It is common for blood pressure to rise as people age, but this is not physiologically normal or healthy; it is sometimes considered normal by physicians because it is so common. The following is a preliminary program, which can be easily enhanced if it is not working adequately, to lower blood pressure. Of course, if the problem is severe or nonresponsive, medication may be in order. If there are other complicating conditions, other supplements may be helpful.

SUPPLEMENT	A.M.	P.M.
Basic Multiple Formula	3	3
Arginine 500 mg	2	2
Coenzyme Q_{10} 100 mg		1
EPA fish oil capsules, 1,000 mg	2	2
Garlic, deodorized, 500 mg	1	1
GLA 240 mg (from borage oil)		1
Magnesium aspartate 200 mg	1	1
Pyridoxine (B_6) 250 mg		1
Taurine 500 mg	2	2
Vitamin C 1,000 mg	3	3
Vitamin E 400 IU natural, mixed	1	1

Immune Enhancement

The immune system is a complex interaction of organs (liver, spleen, lymph nodes, and intestines), white blood cells (B-cells; T-cells; natural killer cells) that produce antibodies or engulf invaders, hormones, and regulatory substances (interleukins; prostaglandins; interferon) that combine to protect us from infections and abnormal cells such as cancer. Numerous health problems result from reduced or altered immunity, especially as people age and become less resistant to infections. Many nutrients, indeed almost all of them, help with maintaining and restoring immunity. Some of the more specific ones can help with a variety of immune system disorders.

Enhanced immunity does not necessarily mean an uncontrolled increase in immune activity. Some conditions of altered immunity are the result of *autoimmunity,* where the immune cells and antibodies attack your own tissues and organs. When you hear that a nutrient increases immunity, you do not have to worry that it might increase the activity of an autoimmune disease. What it will do is to help rebalance the immune activity. Restoring immune balance will lessen the likelihood that your immune system will go awry and attack normal tissues. Many dietary supplements help restore this balance, and many of them help to fight off viruses, bacteria, fungi, and cancer cells. The goal of treatment is to support and normalize all the components of the immune system. These supplements work best if combined with a healthy diet, exercise, and stress management programs. Stress is known to harm the immune system, so learn how to relax while you do other things to help.

SUPPLEMENT	A.M.	P.M.
Basic Multiple Formula	3	3
Echinacea 250 mg (Standardized)	1	1
GLA 240 mg (from borage oil)	1	
L-Arginine 500 mg	2	2
L-Glutamine 500 mg	2	2
Magnesium aspartate 200 mg	1	
Siberian ginseng 200 mg	1	1
Transfer factor 200 mg	2	2
Vitamin C 1,000 mg	3	3
Vitamin E 400 IU natural, mixed	1	1

Menopause

Menopause is the absence of the menstrual cycle for one year, although the symptoms of menopause often occur before the periods are completely finished and for some time thereafter. As the function of the ovaries declines gradually, the entire time frame may be from a few years before the end of the menstrual cycles to some years afterward. Menopause generally happens between the ages of 48 and 52, but it may be as early as forty or as late as the late fifties. It also happens when the ovaries are removed surgically. This is most commonly done as part of a total hysterectomy or when there is ovarian cancer.

The menopausal transition is normal, but symptoms may not be. In other cultures with different dietary habits, women may not have any symptoms at all. However, in Western cultures symptoms are very common although some women make the transition with relative ease. In addition to hot flashes and night sweats, symptoms may include depression, mood swings, irritability, and vaginal dryness.

One of the most important dietary choices you can make to help with menopausal symptoms is to include more soy products in your diet. This means more tofu, soy milk, tempeh, and soy nuts. Soy foods are rich in isoflavones called genistein and daidzein. These have mild estrogenic properties that help with menopause (but not any of the side effects of estrogen replacement therapy).

I also recommend supplements of ipriflavone, a modified isoflavone that has been shown to build bone density and reverse osteoporosis—the bone loss that accelerates after menopause. In addition to those listed in the chart, other helpful supplements include the hormones progesterone (natural, not the more common synthetic derivatives) and DHEA, and the herbs Vitex agnuscastus and dong quai. You may respond better to one or more of these supplements, and you have to find the combination that works for you, but these are the ones I have found most effective in my medical practice.

SUPPLEMENT	A.M.	P.M.
Basic Multiple Formula	3	3
Bioflavonoid mix 1,000 mg	1	1
Black cohosh 40 mg	2	2
Flaxseed oil, Tbsp		1–2
GLA 240 mg (from borage oil)	1	
Ipriflavone 300 mg	1	1
Magnesium aspartate 200 mg		1
Vitamin C 1,000 mg	2	2
Vitamin E 400 IU natural, mixed	1	1

Osteoporosis

Bones are dynamic living tissues, containing calcium, magnesium, phosphorus, and other minerals, and they are constantly being re-formed through a balance of mineral deposits and mineral loss. This takes place through a complex interaction of bone-forming cells called osteoblasts and bone-resorbing cells called osteoclasts, but with aging the balance shifts toward loss of bone minerals and bone strength.

After the age of thirty to thirty-five, bone loss, or demineralization, in both men and women, is about 1 percent a year. After menopause, the rate of bone loss in women accelerates to about 3 percent a year. You can see that, at this rate, five or seven years after menopause women will have lost up to 20 percent of their bone density.

Twenty-five to thirty million Americans have osteoporosis, and that number is expected to increase significantly in the next twenty years. The overwhelming majority of them are women, but men also have osteoporosis as they also lose bone every year. (Men usually do not have osteoporosis as early as women do because they start with a higher bone density before the demineralization begins.) As the number of aging Americans increases, it is important to do something to prevent and treat bone loss.

This thinning or weakening of the skeleton leads to bone fractures, which is often the first outward sign that a problem exists. Sometimes the fracture appears to be the result of a fall, when in fact the fracture of the severely weakened hip was the cause of the fall, not the other way around. The most common sites of fracture are the hip, the spine, and the wrist.

Weight-bearing exercise is essential to the prevention of osteoporosis. It appears that the impact or stress on the bones increases bone density when combined with proper diet and other healthy habits. The diet is also of critical importance. Milk is not a cure for osteoporosis. It appears from population studies that milk also does nothing to prevent osteoporosis. This is contrary to the popular myth fostered by the milk industry. Countries with the highest milk consumption have the highest rates of osteoporosis and hip fracture. After weaning, milk is not a very healthy food.

Dietary habits that increase bone loss are consumption of high amounts of protein (especially animal protein), phosphorus (found in milk, meat, and especially sodas), sugar, caffeine, and alcohol. Changing this to a mostly vegetarian diet of unprocessed foods is very likely to help prevent osteoporosis (and many other health problems).

Hormone replacement therapy with estrogens has been shown to retard bone loss, but not to actually build bone (whereas supplements of natural progesterone can build up bone density). Ipriflavone supplements have been shown to both retard bone loss and increase bone density better than estrogens.

In addition, I recommend about 1,000 mg of calcium and extra vitamin D. For women who want to take hormone replacement therapy, I strongly suggest avoiding Premarin and Provera, the most common supplements, and take natural estrogens in the proper balance, and natural progesterone. I suggest that you have medical advice on this from a physician familiar with natural hormones and nutritional therapy.

SUPPLEMENT	A.M.	P.M.
Basic Multiple Formula	3	3
Bioflavonoid mix 1,000 mg	1	1
Calcium citrate 250 mg	1	1
Flaxseed oil, Tbsp		1–2
GLA 240 mg (from borage oil)	1	
Ipriflavone 300 mg	1	1
Magnesium aspartate 200 mg		1
Vitamin C 1,000 mg	2	2
Vitamin D 400 IU	1	
Vitamin E 400 IU natural, mixed	1	1

Premenstrual Syndrome (PMS)

Premenstrual symptoms range from mild to severe, and they include bloating, cramps, headaches, fluid retention, depression, lower back pain, abdominal pressure, sugar cravings, anxiety, irritability, breast tenderness, acne, and mood swings. Some of these symptoms may also occur during the menstrual period, especially cramps, and they are often controlled by the same supplements.

For both premenstrual and menstrual symptoms, in addition to the dietary supplement program, you may need supplements of *natural progesterone.* This is the hormone (produced primarily by the ovaries, but also by the adrenal glands), that supports pregnancy and also helps to maintain and increase bone density. It also counteracts excessive estrogen stimulation.

Natural progesterone (as opposed to synthetic "progestins" such as Provera) has no side effects and it regulates many different functions. It is particularly important to menopausal women to help *increase* bone density and managing some menopausal symptoms. (Synthetic progestins are different, and have a number of side effects.) Progesterone deficiency is common, and supplements of natural progesterone can be taken either orally or as a skin cream, and they are free of side effects. It is wise to have a gynecological examination before proceeding with progesterone treatment.

In addition to the herbs *Vitex agnuscastus,* and dong quai, the following supplements are those most commonly helpful with both premenstrual syndrome and menstrual symptoms:

SUPPLEMENT	A.M.	P.M.
Basic Multiple Formula	3	3
EPA 1,000 mg, or	2	2
Flaxseed oil, Tbsp		1–2
GLA 240 mg (from borage oil)	1	
Magnesium aspartate 200 mg	1	1
Pyridoxine (B_6) 250 mg	1	
Vitamin C 1,000 mg	2	2
Vitamin E 400 IU natural mixed		1

Prostate Enlargement

Prostate enlargement (benign prostatic hypertrophy or BPH) is a common affliction in men as they age. The prostate gland sits beneath the bladder and surrounds the urethra, the outflow channel for urine. Symptoms of enlargement include difficulty starting or stopping urination, frequent urination, urination at night, slow urine flow, and a frequent sense of urgency to urinate. Surgery to remove some of the prostate tissue is commonly performed if the symptoms become severe enough, and some new procedures using lasers or microwaves can be very effective with fewer side effects.

There are many healthy approaches to managing prostate enlargement. If the symptoms are not severe, there is no risk from trying the alternatives to surgery. The new medication for BPH, finasteride, or Proscar, is not as effective as the herbs and other dietary supplements, and it has potential side effects. Many patients claim that adding pumpkin seeds to their diet helped them. Pumpkin seeds contain zinc and essential fatty acids that may help the condition. The following program of supplements is what I recommend for management of prostate problems:

SUPPLEMENT	A.M.	P.M.
Basic Multiple Formula	3	3
GLA 240 mg (from borage oil)	1	
Magnesium aspartate 200 mg	1	1
Nettle (Urtica dioica) standardized 125 mg	1	1
Pygeum africanum 25 mg	1	1
Saw palmetto standardized 160 mg	1	1
Vitamin C 1,000 mg	3	3
Vitamin E 400 IU natural, mixed	1	1
Zinc 50 mg	1	

Sexual Dysfunction

The interest and ability to partake in satisfying sexual relations is an important part of living, even well into advanced years. It is also an important part of loving relationships. However, there are many causes of sexual dysfunction (loss of interest or ability to take part in sex). This is sometimes called impotence in men.

Any serious medical condition, sexually transmitted diseases, depression or other psychological disorders, fatigue, overwork, or simply lack of adequate sleep can all lead to loss of libido (interest in sex) or ability. Hardening of the arteries to the pelvic organs may be a direct cause of sexual dysfunction. Viagra works by affecting nitric oxide levels, which then affect local circulation, but the same effect may be achieved with supplements of arginine. Of course, loss of interest or ability may also result from relationship problems.

Many poor health habits lead to deterioration of numerous bodily functions, and sexuality is particularly vulnerable. Smoking, obesity, high stress, lack of exercise, fatty acid imbalance (which affects hormones), and alcohol consumption are examples. Chronic problems such as candidiasis, hypoglycemia, allergies, and chronic fatigue syndrome can all lead to sexual dysfunction.

Almost any health-enhancing program of diet and exercise with basic dietary supplements can help the situation. It is also important to deal first with known medical and psychological problems. Even some of these may be helped with nutrition and dietary supplements. Remember to start by changing those harmful life habits. They will not only begin to improve your love life; they will also help to prevent the chronic and lethal degenerative diseases. An initial dietary supplement program that is likely to help is the following:

SUPPLEMENT	A.M.	P.M.
Basic Multiple Formula	3	3
Arginine 500 mg	2	2
Coenzyme Q_{10} *100 mg*	1	
DHEA 5–25 mg (women–men)	1	
Ginkgo biloba *extract 60 mg*	1	1
GLA 240 mg (as borage oil)	1	
Magnesium aspartate 200 mg	1	1
Vitamin C 1,000 mg	2	2
Vitamin E 400 IU natural mixed	1	1

If the cause of sexual dysfunction is diabetes, heart disease, or hormonal imbalances, this program is likely to provide some help, but it is only the beginning. There are more vigorous programs for these conditions that may also help restore your sexuality and help you regain your love life.

For women with specific hormonal needs, natural progesterone supplements or natural estrogens may be valuable. For men, testosterone replacement is often part of a total program. (Even for women, there are therapeutic uses of testosterone in the treatment of heart disease and sexual dysfunction.) Hormonal supplementation with DHEA (dehydroepiandrosterone) is often of benefit to both men and women. Some of these hormones are prescription medications, but not all. A growing number of medical doctors are interested in these modern treatments and can provide good advice on both the prescription and nonprescription doses. For vascular causes of sexual dysfunction in both men and women, EDTA chelation therapy may provide great benefit, as it improves circulation to the pelvic organs.

Notes on Your Health Program

As you can see, these examples of treatment programs have many similarities. This is because many of the same supplements help a variety of health problems. Also, sometimes, different supplements help the same problem, and what works will vary from one person to another.

Your response to herbs and flavonoids may be quite different from the response of your neighbor, or even that of another family member. This is the nature of biochemical individuality. Fortunately, there are also a lot of similarities among people, and this allows physicians to learn what to do for one person from our experience with another. However, the differences between people may require adjusting what we learn and adapting it for the individual. This is part of the art of healing.

These programs are useful starting points for your own needs, or if you are a physician, they can be used as foundations for developing treatment programs for your patients. You do not have to try everything at once. Whether you are just beginning a dietary supplement health program, or if you are a physician just starting in the field, you will benefit by trying only one or a few supplements and adding new ones as you become more familiar with the substances.

You know your body's individual responses better than anyone else, in some ways even better than your health practitioner, and you have to use that information to create your own health or to help your health practitioner guide you. If your practitioners are unfamiliar with this information about dietary supplements, you can help them begin to understand it by giving them this book. This will help you to become a partner in your health care.

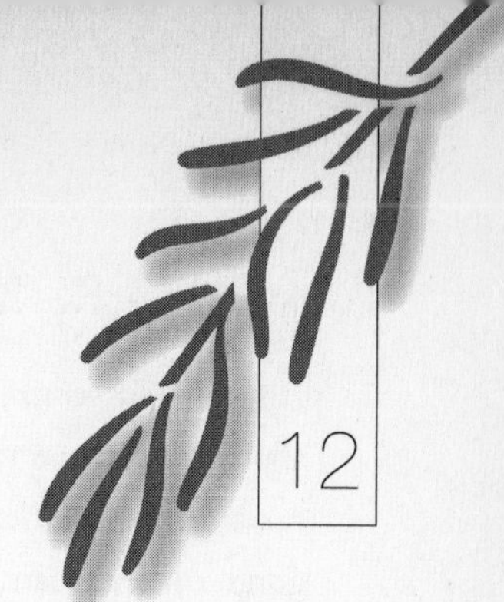

12

My Personal Prevention Program

I HAVE BEEN TAKING dietary supplements for thirty years. Before I started in 1970, I had the same attitude most doctors had then, as many still do today, that if you follow a balanced diet you don't need supplements. As you have seen, this is simply not true (and many doctors, and even dietitians, still do not know what a good diet is). Fortunately, I learned about supplements early in my career—and even more fortunately for me, early in my life.

I now feel as healthy as, or healthier than, I did when I started taking supplements at twenty-five years old. I have virtually no colds, normal weight, good cholesterol levels, no signs of degenerative disease, lots of energy, and a sense of vitality, all of which is unusual in my age group. Part of this is surely due to my healthy, whole-foods, mostly vegetarian diet (I eat no meat or chicken), part to my love of exercise, and some to my genes, but these are certainly enhanced by the supplements that I have taken over the years.

Fanatical or Realistic?

Although it seems to some people almost fanatical that I am so careful about my diet and take so many supplements, it is strange to me that *they* do not think it fanatical to drink sodas, eat potato chips and doughnuts, and gorge on ice cream, candy, steaks, and burgers. And, although my health practices seem fanatical to some, they are clearly beneficial for comprehensive health, medical treatment, and preventive medicine.

To me, living any other way seems extreme. When I watch what other people put in their carts at the supermarket (I go there to buy paper and cleaning products and to the health food store to buy all my groceries), I am always amazed at how much junk they choose. It appears that they don't see the connection between what they choose and the high cost of their health care, or between their choices and how they feel. To me, it is more radical to take a medication or to submit to surgery to make a repair than to follow a healthy lifestyle. This is the realistic choice for anyone who wants to be healthy. Even though there is a genetic component to many diseases, for the chronic degenerative diseases this is almost never as important as the lifestyle choices that you make every day.

A Leaky Valve

When I was a freshman at college, a routine evaluation of all heart murmurs among first-year students revealed that I did not have a benign murmur, as had been told to my family and me all my life. Instead, I learned that I had a truly leaky aortic valve, and the doctors said that I should give up all vigorous exercise (anything more active than golf or chess!). I was told that the condition (aortic insufficiency) would most likely deteriorate with time over the next fifteen to thirty years. The doctors also said that I would most likely develop congestive heart failure as the heart became unable to keep up with the greater pumping needs (always having to send a little extra out to make up for the amount that leaked back into the heart).

At the time of my diagnosis in 1962, I had no reason to doubt the validity of what the doctors were saying. Somehow, though, even accepting the diagnosis (which I have never doubted), I was unable to allow their fears for my future health to follow me into my own life. I continued, with what some doctors considered reckless abandon, to play sports (although I used their excuse notes to escape gym requirements).

Much later in life, I learned that the doctors had wanted to replace my aortic valve with a plastic one, but my parents refused to accept surgery since I was asymptomatic, and they had a healthy skepticism of excess medical treatment. (The technology of valve replacement has improved enormously since that time, so if I ever do need a new valve, the chances of success are much greater now than they were in 1962, and I expect them to continue to improve.)

A Change of Direction

I became interested in vitamin supplements and diet through the influence of a fascinating older Norwegian psychologist/musician/nutritionist, Kaare Bolgen, who convinced me that I hadn't learned everything in medical school. At the time, this was a shocking revelation. I had also developed a healthy skepticism of many medical treatments. I was a hospital resident, training in pathology, and I saw firsthand in the morgue the results of many dangerous lifestyle choices, as well as the overuse of some surgical heart treatments. I had a personal interest in doing the best I could for my heart, and I developed an interest in longevity in spite of my doctors' dire predictions. This interest in true "health care," as opposed to "disease care," was soon translated into my medical practice.

As of this writing, Kaare is more than ninety-two years old, and speaking with him recently I learned that he is still ice-skating regularly and has just finished writing a book. He has been a longtime vegetarian, and he takes numerous dietary supplements, many in large doses.

Since my exposure to the importance of dietary supplements, I have been recommending them for my patients and anyone else who wants to listen, and taking them myself. I have also run marathons, and enjoy running, walking, playing racquetball, long-distance bicycling, in-line skating, and skiing—both cross country and downhill. I eat a whole-foods diet, especially avoiding sugar and margarines, which is mostly vegetarian (no meat or chicken), and I try to keep my stress levels under control.

In the early 1980s, I went to see another cardiologist, Dr. George Sheehan, who was a distance runner himself and a well-known writer on running. His conclusion, after evaluating my heart, was that my earlier doctors were right in their description of what "might" happen, but they had no scientific reason to claim that exercise would bring on heart failure. It might even be the case that exercise would make the situation better. I have since learned that with aortic valve insufficiency, exercise actually can do more good than harm by shortening the resting phase (diastole) of the heartbeat.

Also, the earlier cardiologists did not account for the nutrition and dietary supplements that could help strengthen and protect the heart. Of course, that was in 1962, and there were only a few people who were aware of the relationship between diet, supplements, and disease—I was not one of them.

Through medical school I had the same health habits as my fellow students—burgers, fries, cola, and frequent coffee. I also exercised only periodically and knew nothing of stress control (other than frequent laughter). These are the typical unhealthy habits of young people, but they are now known to lead to serious problems after the resilience of youth is dissipated, and sometimes even earlier. I survived this without observable serious problems, but I continued to have several colds and flus each year.

I now take many supplements, and, as I become older, I am increasing the doses or varieties of those that protect me from the ravages of aging and free-radical damage. I am not suggesting that my own program is right for anyone else, but I am presenting it as an example of a vigorous health-enhancement program that I suspect will keep me healthy well into advanced years. I am always modifying my own intake, based on new knowledge and the availability of new supplements or new forms of supplements.

No one has a way of knowing what will happen in the future, but one of the advantages of a longevity program such as mine is that it also keeps me feeling vigorous and alive in the present. Results in the present are what keep most people on track, and I am no different. As you feel better on your own program, your desire to stay with it will be reinforced.

What I Take

I take my supplements twice every day, and almost never miss a dose. If I miss the morning dose for any reason, I will take them later with my lunch. I vary my intake somewhat from day to day, and I have altered my intake since the first edition of this book. Some of the supplements on the list I now take periodically and then take a break from them. For example, I take carnitine and glutamine several times a week, not daily. I also take echinacea to enhance immunity, but only for a few days several times a month or if I feel that I might be getting a virus (a rare situation these days). I take elderberry extract for the same purpose. I added ginseng to my program—Korean in the morning and Siberian or American in the evening. I now take 100 mg of phosphatidyl serine for memory and 333 mg of lipoic acid as an antioxidant; I reduced my vitamin C slightly because of the mix of other antioxidants I take. Sometimes I take kava kava as a relaxant at bedtime. My personal supplement program consists of the following intake:

SUPPLEMENT	A.M.	P.M.
Basic Multiple Formula	3	3
Bioflavonoid mix 1,000 mg	1	1
Chromium niacinate/picolinate 300 mcg	1	
Coenzyme Q_{10} *200 mg chewable*	1	
Eye nutrients/including bilberry 100 mg	1	1
Folic acid 20 mg	1	
Ginkgo biloba *extract 60 mg*	1	1
Ginseng 200 mg	1	1
GLA 240 mg (borage oil)	1	
L-Carnitine 250 mg	2	2
L-Glutamine 500 mg	2	2
Lipoic acid 333 mg	1	
Lutein 20 mg	1	
Lycopene 10 mg	1	
Magnesium aspartate 200 mg	1	
Melatonin 3 mg		1

Natural carotenoids 25,000 IU	1	
Niacin-inositol 400 mg	1	1
Proanthocyanidins 50 mg mixed	1	1
Pyridoxine (B_6) 250 mg	1	
Quercetin 400 mg	1	1
Saw palmetto/pygeum/nettle combination	1	1
Selenium 200 mcg	1	
Special antioxidant formula	1	1
Vitamin C 1,000 mg	5	5
Vitamin E 400 IU natural mixed	1	1

I take all my supplements after breakfast or supper, except that I take the melatonin at bedtime. I take the saw palmetto extract, pygeum, and nettle, although I have no sign of prostate enlargement, because I believe that in my age group it is good preventive medicine.

I also take some other supplements periodically, or as needed, if I feel stressed or fatigued. I also take three or four capsules of silymarin for liver cleansing on occasion. If I have been very busy and my mind is racing, I might add some calming herbs (valerian, skullcap, passion flower, and hops in a combination), or kava kava to my bedtime dose of melatonin. Sometimes I take an extra coenzyme Q_{10} tablet, or higher doses of L-carnitine, and L-glutamine.

As I learn about new research on dietary supplements and orthomolecular substances, I am always on the lookout for materials that might help both my patients and me enhance our health. In addition to doing things that promote my own health, I believe in setting the example for my patients in exercise, diet, stress reduction, and dietary supplementation. It is much easier to believe professionals who practice what they preach. (Because I only preach what I practice, it is easy for me to set a good example; it does not require any great virtue.) I expect to be setting the example for many years to come.

Science and Medicine

Part of what I am doing is experimental, but that does not mean that it is not documented. Science is an important method of study that always gives us new information and new ways of looking at information. The facts revealed by scientific study are never perfect. Imperfect data must always be used to draw conclusions, but we have to be open to the possibility that later information will change our view and provide new insights into the role of dietary supplements in health care—both treatment and prevention. Although medicine is based in science, it is fundamentally an art, depending on judgment, knowledge of the patient, compassion, and intuition, in addition to the scientific studies.

I do not want to wait for the final scientific word on these safe supplements. They have good research and clinical experience to back them up, and anyway, science never provides the final word—it is a dynamic search for truth that always depends on the current state of our knowledge. Right now, that knowledge says that the wisest approach to health care, along with diet, exercise, and stress management, includes taking dietary supplements.

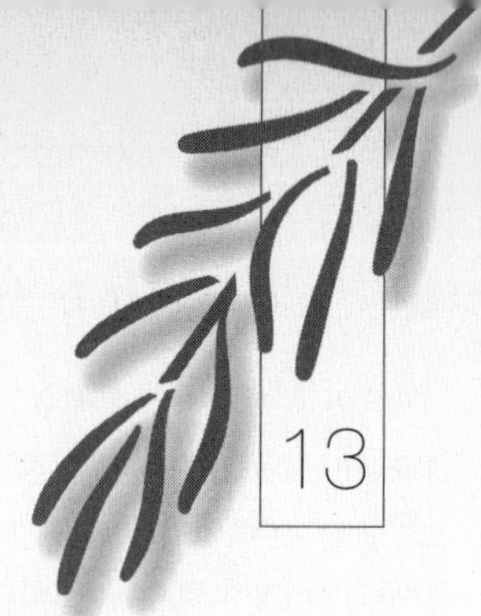

13

Dietary Supplements: Political Pressure Cooker

IN RECENT YEARS, the political and bureaucratic pressures surrounding dietary supplements have exploded with new attempts by the United States Food and Drug Administration (FDA) to restrict the flow of information about them. Through a misguided fear of "snake-oil salesmen" and a mission to promote the development and safety of new drugs, the FDA has been on a vendetta against the dietary supplement industry since early in its history.

This situation in the United States has implications for other countries, because many of them take their regulatory cues from the actions of the FDA. In Norway, for example, doses of supplements beyond the RDA were at first banned, and then the government opened a chain of stores that became the only ones allowed to sell high-dose supplements. In 1994, I had an opportunity to testify at meetings in Great Britain concerning European Economic Community regulations of dietary supplement doses. The issue under discussion at the time concerned the safety of vitamin B_6, and it has been tentatively resolved with no action against reasonable doses of B_6 because the data do not show any toxicity at levels under 500 mg. This is an ongoing struggle in many countries and seems to threaten the status quo wherever anyone wants to take charge of his or her own health care.

Protecting You from Information

The FDA's regulatory efforts are purportedly aimed at protecting the public from misinformation that the marketers of dietary supplements might use to sell their products. It is true that this has happened in the past and is happening, although to a lesser extent, today. However, the issue has come to the fore because in their zeal the FDA is "protecting" the public from accurate information that will do them a world of good.

The truth is, there has been an explosion of new research data showing the value of dietary supplements in almost every sphere of health care. From cancer to heart disease to AIDS to headaches, dietary supplements are being shown to be of value. They are helping people stay off drugs and they are reducing the costs of health care, in terms of both money and undesired side effects.

In spite of official opposition to supplements (from both government agencies and much of mainstream medicine), the public demand for them is growing. In response to this, the FDA has used rule making and legal maneuvering to subvert the intent of the laws that Congress passed designed to increase the flow of nutrition information to the public.

In 1992 and 1993, Congress considered bills that would restrict the ability of the FDA to skirt the intent of the laws. During the hearings held by the Senate Labor and Human Resources Committee in 1993, David Kessler, then commissioner of the FDA, made some erroneous statements about supplements. He also displayed some bottles of dietary supplements that he claimed were "misbranded" because they made health claims.

Any health claims for dietary supplements were against the regulations of the FDA if they were made by supplement manufacturers or distributors, even if they were truthful and not misleading and even if they were the same health claims that other agencies of the U.S. government were making. For example, if the U.S. Public Health Service suggested folic acid supplements for pregnant women, it was illegal for a company marketing folic acid to quote that agency in its promotional literature, saying that folate could prevent birth defects.

The bill then being considered, the Dietary Supplement and Health Education Act (DSHEA), eventually passed despite the vehement opposition of some Congressional protectors of the FDA. However, many of the most important sections of the Senate version of the bill, which would allow the easiest public access to supplement information, were deleted before the bill was passed by the House of Representatives.

I testified at those 1993 Senate hearings and had to depart from my prepared testimony in order to address some of the misinformation presented by the director of the FDA. I then submitted to the committee some written follow-up testimony that included most of the statements that I felt compelled to present ad lib. Although I have seen it many times, I am always surprised when scientific information is misrepresented for political purposes. (For my full Senate testimony, see Appendix 3.)

Since the passage of DSHEA, the FDA has tried to redefine the meaning of the term *disease* in an effort to circumvent the restrictions placed on them by the law. Because structure/function claims are allowed, you can say that chromium is helpful in regulation of blood sugar, or that vitamin E helps circulation. But disease claims are not allowed, so you cannot say that chromium is helpful for diabetes or that vitamin E helps heart disease. In order to extend their reach, the FDA has tried to claim that some abnormal functions are really diseases, when they are only symptoms of diseases. For example, menopause is a normal event, but the FDA is trying to define it as a disease, so supplement manufacturers cannot say that certain herbs can help with the associated symptoms.

The Federal Trade Commission (FTC) has taken up the banner where the FDA has been restricted. They are claiming that they are not bound by DSHEA, and that they can prosecute companies that make claims based on a different level of evidence than that required by DSHEA. All the concerned public groups and members of Congress are following this bureaucratic maneuver very closely to make sure that DSHEA is not undermined. The FTC does not have the capacity to determine what is adequate scientific evidence for health claims. To make their decisions they choose experts, and, having worked with the FTC on other matters, I am not convinced that they choose them in an unbiased manner.

Unfortunately, in spite of the ultimate passage of a watered-down version of the Dietary Supplement Health and Education Act, there are still political, behind-the-scenes maneuverings that make it unclear what will happen with regulation and oversight of dietary supplements by the FDA. The FDA officials and lawyers have been working tirelessly to "interpret" the language of the bill to try to maintain their restriction on availability of supplements and on access to information about them. In 1999, the FDA lost an important court case on label claims. They must now define what they mean by "significant scientific agreement" so that companies can make legitimate claims, and they must allow certain claims. In spite of having lost in court, they still try to make it difficult for people to get this information, and it appears that they are trying to protect drug company interests rather than the public.

If you want to help ensure the continued availability of dietary supplements and your access to information about them, you can contact your representatives in Washington and let them know you want their support for this. You can also support several organizations that, as of 1999, are working toward passage of a revision of the dietary supplement bill. This will surely still be an issue for the next few years. One of these organizations is the American Preventive Medical Association (see Appendix 2), which is working toward more health freedom in many ways. Another is Citizens for Health, a grass-roots organization supporting health freedom.

In 1998, Congress established the National Center for Complementary and Alternative Medicine (NCCAM) at the National Institutes of Health. Formerly, this was only an office, not a center, and did not have as much autonomy to support the research that is so essential for the development of alternative medicine. The budget of the Center has been increased, and it is likely that serious research will now have some of the necessary funding.

Health Endangered in Canada

In Canada, dietary supplement consumers have faced similar problems to those in the U.S. And their regulations may be even worse. In 1995, the Canadian parliament considered a bill (C-7) that would have made it difficult to find any over-the-counter dietary supplements. Because they have an effect on states of health, it was proposed that access to supplements and information about them be restricted.

The bill would have technically criminalized anyone who sold any herbal remedy or natural supplement with stimulant or relaxant properties. Tryptophan is already a prescription drug in Canada, and its price has risen dramatically since losing its over-the-counter status. (It is also available in the U.S. by prescription, at a higher cost than previously.)

Other substances that are harmful to health would have been specifically exempted from coverage by this bill. Thus, Canadians might have been in the ridiculous position of being able to buy nicotine, alcohol, and caffeine freely but not large doses of vitamin C or vitamin E. It can hardly be argued that the main goal of that bill was to protect public health. There would have been an exemption for prescription drugs, which are at least twenty-five hundred times more dangerous than dietary supplements. Canadian associations are still working toward greater freedom of access to supplements and information about them. (See Appendix 2.)

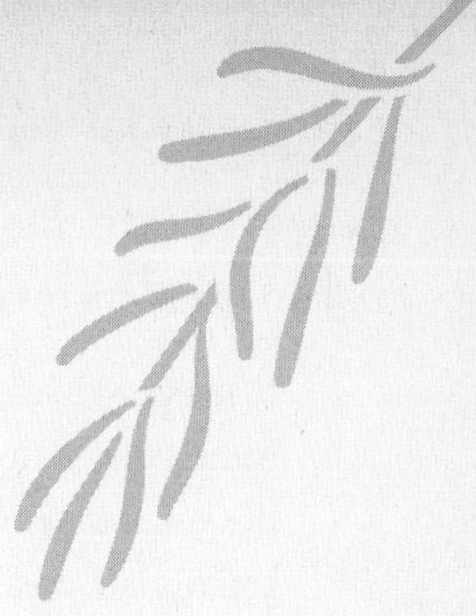

Conclusion

THIS HAS BEEN a brief overview of the use of dietary supplements in health-care and health-oriented medicine. It gives you a good foundation for establishing your own supplement regimen as part of your total health program. If you have serious health problems, you would be wise to seek the advice of a health professional—and wisest to look for one who understands and accepts the value of good health habits and dietary supplements, and is knowledgeable enough to make recommendations. Working together you can plan a total health program for your individual needs.

As you can see, most dietary supplements that are specific nutrients are useful for both prevention and treatment. The herbal supplements are more frequently valuable for treatment of specific health problems but sometimes are also valuable for prevention, stress, or longevity. For example, echinacea and silymarin are helpful for immune enhancement and liver protection if you take them periodically while you are healthy and ginseng helps for coping with stress and immune function. Many herbal products are also helpful in minor acute illnesses or as first-aid treatments.

Try Supplements First

It is clear that many conditions that are treated with drugs should be treated first with a proper total health program and dietary supplements. If the situation is an emergency, then I am all in favor of immediate and appropriate medical or surgical treatments. However, even in these circumstances, nutrients might be the first choice. Recent studies have shown that magnesium infusions for heart attack patients can significantly reduce serious complications and deaths. It can also be a first line of treatment for acute asthma. If health problems do not respond to nutrition, dietary supplements, exercise, and stress reduction, medicine and surgery are still available.

Most health problems are not emergencies. To treat them as though they were chronic, recurrent emergencies, which is the way medicine is often practiced today, is costly, time-consuming, and generally ineffective. It causes many problems, often more than it relieves, and these are sometimes deadly. Side effects of medications kill more people annually than automobile accidents. As noted in chapter 2, side effects of prescription medications fall somewhere between fourth and sixth as a leading cause of death. Unnecessary surgery (for heart disease and other conditions) has significant mortality, while it also drives up health-care costs. Bypass surgery is the ninth leading cause of death. This approach to health care also takes the power and responsibility for your health out of your control.

Your Personal Power for Health

The intensity of debate in government circles that revolves around solving the "health care crisis" is misguided, misinformed, and misnamed. It has nothing to do with health, but is really an effort to find ways to pay for the excess disease care that too many Americans need. They need this extra care because they do not take proper care of their personal health. You can personally do more than the entire government toward solving the health crisis and the high cost of medical care—simply by taking care of yourself and decreasing your own costs of health care.

While the government can do little to solve the larger health crisis, there is much that you can do for yourself that will have a far greater impact on your own health than any government program. It is a mistake to think that the government is honestly interested in health when they allow fast-food companies to provide the food services at schools, and when high government officials set the wrong example by having photo ops of themselves in the local burger-fries-and-a-shake joint, even if they jog to get there.

You do not have to accept this situation. Ultimately, you are responsible for your own health. I once saw a mock ad in a health magazine that said, "Wanted: Reformers; not of the government but of themselves." It must begin with you.

If you are ill or just not feeling up to par, you should know that *in most circumstances you have the power to create your own health.* You can do it with simple lifestyle changes and dietary supplements. If you need education and professional advice to begin your path to self-determined health, you have already started by reading this book.

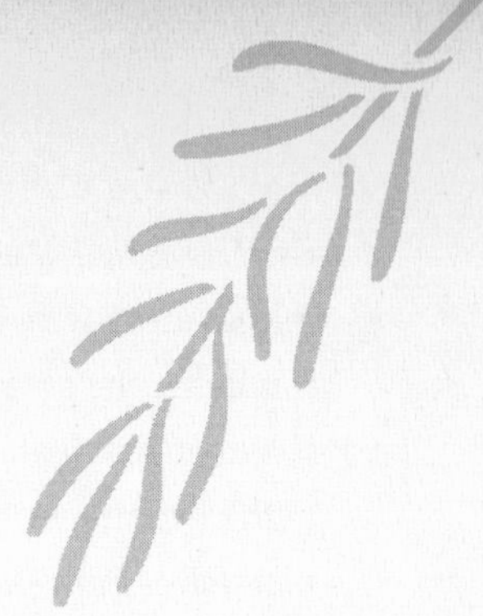

List of Abbreviations

A4M	American Academy of Anti-Aging Medicine
AAEM	American Academy of Environmental Medicine
AANP	American Association of Naturopathic Physicians
ACAM	American College for Advancement in Medicine
AHMA	American Holistic Medical Association
AIDS	Acquired immune deficiency syndrome
ALA	Alpha-lipoic acid
APMA	American Preventive Medical Association
ATP	Adenosine triphosphate
BPH	Benign prostatic hypertrophy
CCAM	Center for Complementary and Alternative Medicine (NIH)
CDC	Centers for Disease Control and Prevention
CFIDS	Chronic fatigue immune deficiency syndrome
CN	Certified Nutritionist
CoQ_{10}	Coenzyme Q_{10}
CSPI	Center for Science in the Public Interest

DDT	Dichlorodiphenyl trichloroethane
DGL	Deglycyrrhizinated licorice
DHA	Docosahexaenoic acid
DHEA	Dehydroepiandrosterone
DLPA	DL-phenylalanine
DMG	Dimethyl glycine
DNA	Deoxyribonucleic acid
DV	Daily values
EFA	Essential fatty acids
EMS	Eosinophilia myalgia syndrome
EPA	Eicosapentaenoic acid; Environmental Protection Agency
FDA	(United States) Food and Drug Administration
GABA	Gamma-aminobutyric acid
GLA	Gamma-linolenic acid
GMP	Good Manufacturing Practices
GTF	Glucose tolerance factor
HDL	High-density lipoprotein
LDL	Low-density lipoprotein
LPA	L-phenylalanine
MD	Doctor of Medicine
MHMR	My Health/My Rights (Canada)
MSG	Monosodium glutamate
ND	Doctor of Naturopathy
NLEA	Nutrition Labeling and Education Act
NSAIDs	Nonsteroidal anti-inflammatory drugs
OTC	Over-the-counter
PABA	Para-aminobenzoic acid
PAC	Proanthocyanidins
PBS	Public Broadcasting System
PGE_1	Prostaglandin E_1
PMS	Premenstrual syndrome
PSHW	Physicians and Scientists for a Healthy World
RD	Registered Dietitian
RDA	Recommended Dietary Allowances

RNA	Ribonucleic acid
SOD	Superoxide dismutase
SOMA	Society for Orthomolecular Medicine of America
T_3	Triiodothyronine (thyroid hormone)
T_4	Thyroxine (thyroid hormone)
USDA	United States Department of Agriculture

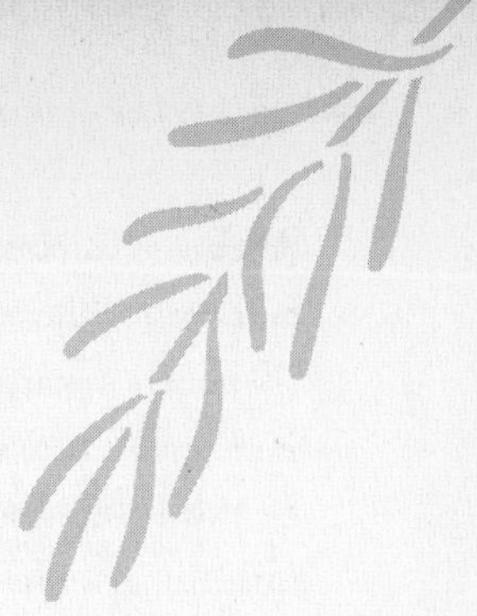

Appendix 1
Dietary Allowances

Recommended Dietary Allowances

RDA, USRDA, RDI, DRI, AND RSAI

The Recommended Dietary Allowances (RDA) were established by the Food and Nutrition Board of the National Research Council–National Academy of Sciences and revised as of 1989. They were designed to prevent deficiency diseases in most healthy people. From them, the FDA derived a different set of values called the "USRDA" for purposes of labeling foods. Updates of these recommendations became the RDI (Reference Daily Intake), and more recently, in 1997, the DRI (Dietary Reference Intake) for the purpose of food labels. However, the deficiency diseases that these nutrients prevent, such as scurvy, pellagra, and beriberi, are not the problems of the industrialized world, and these numbers become somewhat irrelevant in efforts to promote optimal health and avoid chronic, degenerative diseases and cancer.

This table is a combination of the RDAs and the RDIs, or in some cases the RSAI—yet another figure called the "Recommended Safe and

Adequate Intake," which you might consider a preliminary recommended amount for those nutrients for which the standard has not been decided. (Numbers in parentheses mean that different reference tables have different numbers.) There is also a "Daily Value" (or DV; see below). Believe it or not, all this is supposed to make it easier for the layperson to understand the nutritional value of her or his food selections. The amounts listed are derived from FDA tables, *Modern Nutrition in Health and Disease* (Shils, et al., ed.), and *Nutritional Biochemistry and Metabolism* (Linder, ed.).

*Vitamin A (& beta-carotene)**	*5,000/4,000*	*IU*
Vitamin C	*60*	*mg*
Vitamin D	*200 (400)*	*IU*
*Vitamin E**	*15/12 (30)*	*IU*
*Vitamin K**	*80/65*	*mcg*
*Thiamin (B_1)**	*1.5/1.1*	*mg*
*Riboflavin (B_2)**	*1.7/1.3*	*mg*
*Niacin (& niacinamide; B_3)**	*20/15*	*mg*
*Pyridoxine (B_6)**	*2.0/1.6*	*mg*
*Folate (folic acid)**	*200/180 (400)*	*mcg*
Cobalamin (B_{12})	*2 (6)*	*mcg*
Biotin	*100 (300)*	*mcg*
Pantothenic acid (B_5)	*10*	*mg*
Calcium	*800 (1,000)*	*mg*
*Iron**	*10/15 (18)*	*mg*
Phosphorus	*800 (1,000)*	*mg*
Iodine	*150*	*mcg*
*Magnesium**	*350/280 (420/320)*	*mg*
Zinc	*15/12 (15)*	*mg*
Copper	*2-3*	*mg*
Sodium	*2,500*	*mg*
Potassium	*2,500*	*mg*
*Selenium**	*70/55*	*mcg*

*Second value is for women.

Daily Values

On food and supplement labels, you will see nutrients listed as "Percent Daily Value" (on the label as %DV), or the relative amount of that nutrient in a portion of food, compared to the "Daily Value," yet another standard of dietary needs. This "DV" amount is different from the RDI.

Vitamin A (& beta-carotene)	5,000	*IU*
Vitamin C	60	*mg*
Vitamin D	400	*IU*
Vitamin E	30	*IU*
Thiamin (B_1)	1.5	*mg*
Riboflavin (B_2)	1.7	*mg*
Niacin (& niacinamide; B_3)	20	*mg*
Pyridoxine (B_6)	2.0	*mg*
Folate (folic acid)	400	*mcg*
Cobalamin (B_{12})	6.0	*mcg*
Biotin	0.3	*mg*
Pantothenic acid (B_5)	10	*mg*
Calcium	1,000	*mg*
Iron	18	*mg*
Phosphorus	1,000	*mg*
Iodine	150	*mcg*
Magnesium	400	*mg*
Zinc	15	*mg*
Copper	2	*mg*
Sodium	2,500	*mg*
Potassium	4,000	*mg*

There are no Daily Values for other nutrients, such as vitamin K, manganese, selenium and chromium, but this does not mean they are unimportant.

Healthy Dietary Allowances

My own recommendations of nutrient levels for basic health are clearly different from the RDA levels and the Daily Values. They include both food sources and extra amounts derived from dietary supplements. The levels for some of these nutrients are higher than the amounts found in any single multivitamin/mineral combination, so in addition to food and a multi you will need to take some other supplements to fill in the difference. The amounts of vitamin C and folic acid are difficult to get from food alone, but they are not impossible with a diet of mostly fresh fruits and vegetables, whole grains, and beans. For example, asparagus has 160 mcg of folic acid per cup and one avocado about 124 mcg, while liver (although I do not recommend it) has about 1,000 mcg per pound, so you can see that these levels are not impossible to achieve. One papaya has about 187 mg of vitamin C (and only 117 calories), a cup of black currants has 200 mg with only 71 calories, and one cup of broccoli has 82 mg for only 24 calories. You can see that if you choose foods that are "nutrient dense" you will get high levels of nutrients, but you can also achieve these amounts with supplements.

For basic preventive medicine, free-radical protection, and health enhancement I recommend:

Vitamin A (including carotenes)	*25,000*	*IU*
Vitamin C	*4,000*	*mg*
Vitamin D	*400*	*IU*
Vitamin E	*400*	*IU*
Thiamin (B_1)	*100*	*mg*
Riboflavin (B_2)	*50*	*mg*
Niacin (& niacinamide; B_3*)*	*150*	*mg*
Pyridoxine (B_6)	*100*	*mg*
Folate (folic acid)	*2,000*	*mcg*
Cobalamin (B_{12})	*1000*	*mcg*
Biotin	*300*	*mcg*
Pantothenic acid (B_5)	*100*	*mg*
Calcium	*500*	*mg*
Iron	*18*	*mg*

Phosphorus	*1,000 mg*
Iodine	*150 mcg*
Magnesium	*500 mg*
Zinc	*30 mg*
Copper	*3 mg*
Sodium	*500–1,000 mg*
Potassium	*4,000 mg*

Notice that my recommended level for sodium (salt) is *lower* than the DV. It is more a reflection of need than the DV, since excess sodium is unhealthy. The DV is based, in part, on what people are actually getting from food, rather than what is ideal for health. Since consumption of salt is usually so high (5,000–13,000 mg daily!), the DV for sodium is actually above what you really need. (It seems that the people who set these standards are reluctant to tell people how poor their food choices really are.)

My recommendation for calcium is also lower than the RDA. This is predicated on your following a healthier diet than the one common in the United States and many other industrialized countries. If you eat too much protein (especially animal protein), caffeine, sugar, salt, and sodas, then you will very likely need more calcium. You may also need more calcium if you lead a sedentary lifestyle, although more dietary calcium is no substitute for weight-bearing exercise, such as walking or jogging, if maintaining bone density is one of your goals. If you have adequate magnesium nutrition, it is probably quite safe to take extra calcium.

Older standards suggested getting twice as much calcium as magnesium. This was based in part on the ratio of the two minerals in the blood, and does not necessarily reflect dietary needs. Variations in absorption, utilization, and the physiology of the two minerals make the blood levels unreliable figures for determining dietary needs.

Magnesium deficiencies are quite common, marginal deficiencies are difficult to detect, and long-term consequences of low magnesium intake are quite serious. They include neurologic, heart, and kidney diseases. For these reasons I recommend at least as much magnesium as calcium. High calcium intake also increases the need for magnesium.

A healthy diet naturally contains a lot of potassium—well over 4,000 mg daily, because vegetables, fruits, whole grains, and beans are very rich in potassium. However, people taking certain diuretics or those eating a large amount of sodium may need potassium supplements, and the typical American diet is relatively poor in potassium as well as being high in sodium.

Appendix 2

Resources

IF YOU NEED FURTHER ADVICE from a health- or nutrition-oriented professional, there is a growing body of physicians who can help you. The number of medical doctors interested in this field is increasing rapidly. The membership in the American College for Advancement in Medicine, for example, has grown to well above 1,100 members as of 1999 (more than 400 above the number in 1996), and most of the members are experienced in dietary supplements. Members of the American Holistic Medical Association and the American Academy of Environmental Medicine also often have interest in and knowledge of this field. In addition, there are many naturopathic physicians (ND) and certified nutritionists (CN) who may be able to help you.

Not surprisingly, many health food store managers have a lot of information on the value of dietary supplements (but not all of them have completely accurate information). Unfortunately, because of the legal-political situation, even if they are knowledgeable they have to be very circumspect in what information they give out. Sometimes they are only willing to recommend books or articles because even any accurate information they give out may be considered mislabeling by the FDA.

As the political situation is changing, you may find increasing information available through many sources. Structure/function claims are now allowed, meaning that supplement manufacturers and health food stores can inform you that coenzyme Q_{10} helps heart function, and chromium contributes to sugar regulation, that St. John's wort affects mood, and saw palmetto helps the urinary tract. But they cannot tell you that coQ_{10} treats heart failure or hypertension, that chromium treats diabetes, that St. John's wort treats depression, or that saw palmetto treats benign prostate enlargement, even though all these are true.

You can do much further reading, whether you are educating yourself for your own health, or if you are a professional looking to help your patients. Many books written by experienced professionals give practical guidelines and background information. This Appendix is only a partial listing of the books that I recommend. Each one will give many other sources if you wish to pursue more intense study. Some of the books are older and may be out of print, but they will usually be available in the library. They contain valuable background information and further references.

No one book has all the answers and often the books will disagree with each other on some points, but in general there is wide agreement about the value of different dietary supplements. I don't endorse everything that all these books claim, but overall the information is valuable. Whatever you read, make sure you apply some of your own common sense to the material before accepting it. If you see health practitioners for guidance (whether medical doctors, naturopaths, acupuncturists, chiropractors, nutritionists, or others), be sure to ask questions in order to be fully informed about your treatment.

Sources of Supplements

You can find good-quality supplements at health food stores, some nutritionally oriented pharmacies, and from the offices of nutritionally oriented practitioners. I recommend two different mail-order sources for their reliability, quality, and price. Both are available at Web sites on the Internet or by phone and fax.

QCI Nutritionals (1-888-922-4848 or 603-878-1561), or on the Internet at www.qcinutritionals.com.

Willner Chemists (1-800-633-1106) or on the Internet at www.willner.com.

General Books

Steve Austin, N.D., and Cathy Hitchcock, M.S.W.
Breast Cancer: What You Should Know (but May Not Be Told) About Prevention, Diagnosis, and Treatment

James Balch, M.D., and Phyllis Balch, C.N.
Prescription for Nutritional Healing

Jeffrey Bland, Ph.D.
Your Health Under Siege, Using Nutrition to Fight Back

Harold Bloomfield, M.D.
Healing Anxiety with Herbs

Arline and Harold Brecher
Forty-Something Forever

Kenneth Bock, M.D.
The Road to Immunity

Peter Breggin, M.D.
Toxic Psychiatry

James P. Carter, M.D., Dr.P.H.
Racketeering in Medicine: The Suppression of Alternatives

Emmanuel Cheraskin, M.D., D.M.D.
The Vitamin C Connection
Diet and Disease
Psychodietetics
New Hope for Incurable Diseases
Predictive Medicine
Vitamin C: Who Needs It?

Norman Cousins

Anatomy of an Illness

The Healing Heart

Head First

Elmer Cranton, M.D.

Bypassing Bypass: The New Technique of Chelation Therapy

William G. Crook, M.D.

The Yeast Connection

Udo Erasmus

Fats That Heal, Fats That Kill

Rebecca Flynn, M.S., and Mark Roest

Your Guide to Standardized Herbal Products

Alan Gaby, M.D.

B_6, The Natural Healer

Preventing and Reversing Osteoporosis

Abram Hoffer, M.D., Ph.D.

Nutrients to Age Without Senility

Orthomolecular Nutrition

Beatrice Trum Hunter

Consumer Beware! Your Food and What's Been Done to It

The Mirage of Safety: Food Additives and Federal Policy

The Great Nutrition Robbery

Food Additives and Your Health

Richard Kunin, M.D.

Mega-Nutrition

Michael Murray, N.D.

Natural Alternatives to Prozac

The Healing Power of Herbs

Encyclopedia of Nutritional Supplements

Michael Murray, N.D., and Joseph Pizzorno, N.D.

A Textbook of Natural Medicine

Encyclopedia of Natural Medicine

Richard Passwater, Ph.D.

Supernutrition

Supernutrition for a Healthy Heart

Linus Pauling, Ph.D.

Vitamin C and the Common Cold

Vitamin C, the Common Cold, and the Flu

Cancer and Vitamin C

How to Live Longer and Feel Better

Patrick Quillin, Ph.D., R.D.

Healing Nutrients

Beating Cancer with Nutrition

John Robbins

Diet for a New America

Rodale Press (Bill Gottlieb, editor)

New Choices in Natural Healing

Donald Rudin, M.D., and Clara Felix

The Omega-3 Phenomenon

Judy Shabert, M.D., R.D., and Nancy Ehrlich

The Ultimate Nutrient: Glutamine

Charles B. Simone, M.D.

Cancer and Nutrition

Irwin Stone

The Healing Factor: Vitamin C Against Disease

Martin J. Walker

Dirty Medicine: Science, Big Business and the Assault on Natural Health Care

Julian Whitaker, M.D.

Reversing Heart Disease

Reversing Diabetes

Reversing Health Risks

Is Heart Surgery Necessary?

Jonathan Wright, M.D.

Dr. Wright's Book of Nutritional Therapy

Dr. Wright's Guide to Healing with Nutrition

Periodicals/Newsletters

Dr. Michael Janson's Healthy Living, Michael Janson, M.D., editor, Vitality Now!, P.O. Box 384, Greenville, NH, 03048, 603-878-2256 (Also available through QCI Nutritionals, 888-922-4848)

Health and Healing Newsletter, Julian Whitaker, M.D., editor, Phillips Publishing, telephone: 800-777-5005 or 301-424-3700

Health Notes Online, Skye Lininger, D.C., publisher; online and at health food stores

Natural Health

Vegetarian Journal (Vegetarian Resource Group)

Vegetarian Times

Canadian Periodicals

The above magazines are available in Canada, but there are also two magazines that are published in Canada:

Alive, Canadian Journal of Health and Nutrition
at health food stores

Health Naturally, Canada's Self-Health Care Magazine
by subscription or through magazine and health food stores

On-Line Internet Resources

Health data can be retrieved from many computer network sources on the Internet. The following deal with many of the issues presented in this book. The list includes resources for research into the medical literature. You can also look up my own sites on the Internet.

Dr. Janson's Web Sites:

www.drjanson.com. Look for updates on health and medicine, information about Dr. Janson's writing, lectures, and medical practice, and see answers to health questions on the "Ask Dr. J." page. Submit your own questions, and if the questions are of general interest the answers may be posted on the site.

www.healthy.net/janson. This is Dr. Janson's other site, hosted by Health World Online.

American College for Advancement in Medicine (www.acam.org)

ACAM provides a site for physicians and the public. You can locate a practitioner in your area on their Web site, and also find more information about many alternatives in medicine and innovative therapies.

Health World Online (www.healthy.net)

This site is a comprehensive resource for health-related information. You can find experts and libraries of information, excerpts from books and articles, products, and more.

Compuserve Natural Medicine Forum (GO NATMED)

On-line discussions of many health issues and dietary supplements. Extensive library of articles on politics, dietary supplements, nutrition, medical conditions, nutrition software programs, herbs, and other healing methods. For information on Compuserve membership and to receive the free software, call 800-848-8199.

Dr. Elmer Cranton's Web Site (www.drcranton.com)

Dr. Cranton is an experienced physician in nutrition, orthomolecular medicine and chelation therapy. He has edited the *Journal of Holistic Medicine* and the *Journal of Advancement in Medicine,* is the author of *Bypassing Bypass,* and has an informative web site.

The Vitamin C Foundation (www.vitamincfoundation.org)

Extensive information about vitamin C research.

Organic Consumers Association (www.purefood.org)

The Organic Consumers Association is working to maintain organic food standards, and against genetically modified foods and seeds being introduced into the marketplace without extensive further study on safety. They are against any introduction of these foods without complete disclosure through labeling of the products for the consumer. Related sites: Mothers for Natural Law (*www.safe-food.org*); Alliance for Bio-Integrity (*www.biointegrity.org*).

VERIS Research Information Service (www.veris-online.org)

This is a source of research information on vitamins, especially antioxidants, with a focus on carotenoids and vitamin E. It provides abstracts for health professionals, educators, and the media.

Life Extension Foundation (www.lef.org)

A source of information on dietary supplements.

The Linus Pauling Institute (http://osu.orst.edu/dept/lpi)

Julian Whitaker's Health and Healing Newsletter (www.drwhitaker.com)

Dr. Whitaker provides information every month in his newsletter on alternatives in medicine, much of it dealing with dietary supplements.

National Center for Complementary and Alternative Medicine (www.altmed.od.nih.gov/nccam)

This is the new center that started as the Office of Alternative Medicine. It supports research and dissemination of information about alternative medicine.

PubMed Medline Research of the National Library of Medicine (www.ncbi.nlm.nih.gov/pubmed)

For research into the medical literature, this is a free service available to the public.

American Botanical Council (www.herbalgram.org)

A resource for information about herbs and botanical remedies.

Herb Research Foundation (www.herbs.org)

Another resource for information about the therapeutic value of herbs.

International Coenzyme Q_{10} Association (wwwcsi.unian.it/coenzymeQ)

Resource information on coenzyme Q_{10}, conferences, research reports, summaries for laypeople, and membership information.

USDA Food and Nutrition Information Center (www.nal.usda.gov/fnic)

The Food and Nutrition Information Center (FNIC) provides a large amount of data on dietary habits in the United States plus some research information on dietary supplements, from the National Agricultural Library (NAL), part of the United States Department of Agriculture's Agricultural Research Service (ARS). You can access all of FNIC's resource lists and databases through this site.

Professional Books

Rebecca Flynn, M.S., and Mark Roest

Guide to Standardized Herbal Products

William F. Ganong, M.D.

Review of Medical Physiology, 15th ed.

J. B. Harborne, Editor

The Flavonoids: Advances in Research Since 1986

Frank Katch and William McArdle

Introduction to Nutrition, Exercise and Health, 4th ed.

Stephen A. Levine, Ph.D., and Parris Kidd, Ph.D.

Antioxidant Adaptation: Its Role in Free Radical Pathology

Maria Linder, Ph.D., Editor

Nutritional Biochemistry and Metabolism

Medical Economics Company

PDR® for Herbal Medicines

Robert K. Murray et al.

Harper's Biochemistry, 22nd ed.

Maurice Shils, M.D., Sc.D. et al.

Modern Nutrition in Health and Disease, 8th ed.

Gene A. Spiller, Ph.D.

Current Topics in Nutrition and Disease, Volume 4: Nutritional Pharmacology

Melvin Werbach, M.D.

Nutritional Influences on Illness

Nutritional Influences on Mental Illness

Melvin Werbach, M.D., and Michael Murray, N.D.

Botanical Influences on Illness

Professional Journals and Reviews

Clinical Practice of Alternative Medicine (The Official Journal of the American College for Advancement in Medicine) (formerly the Journal of Advancement in Medicine)

Original and review articles on advances in medical care, chelation therapy, and nutrition. American College for Advancement in Medicine. For subscription telephone: 800-532-3688 or 714-583-7666.

CP Currents

Journal abstracts of worldwide literature on nutrition and preventive medicine in print and on CD. ITServices. For subscription, telephone: 916-483-1085.

Clinical Pearls News

Health letter on current research. Includes many relevant articles from the collection in *CP Currents,* plus interviews with researchers on timely topics in nutrition, health care, and dietary supplements. ITServices, 3301 Alta Arden 32, Sacramento, CA 95285. Telephone: 916-483-1085. Fax: 916-483-1431

Alternative Medicine Review

A compilation and review of the most recent published literature on a wide variety of topics related to natural therapeutics. Thorne Research, 901 Triangle Dr., Sandpoint, ID 83864. Telephone: 800-228-1966. Email: kelly@thorne.com

International Clinical Nutrition Reviews

Review articles and abstracts of the world literature on nutrition and dietary supplements. Integrated Therapies, PTY Ltd, PO Box 370, Manly 2095, NSW, Australia.

Journal of Orthomolecular Medicine

Canadian Schizophrenia Foundation, 16 Florence Avenue, Toronto, Ont, M2N 1E9; Telephone: 416-733-2117. They also have available many professional article reprints on nutrition and vitamin therapy.

Journal of Nutrition & Environmental Medicine (UK)

Carfax Publishing Company, PO Box 25, Abingdon, Oxfordshire, OX14 3UE, UK.

Townsend Letter for Doctors and Patients

911 Tyler St., Port Townsend, WA 98368. Telephone: 360-385-6021. Fax: 360-385-0699. Email: cp@olympus.net. Web site: *www.tldp.com.*

Planta Medica
Alternative and Complementary Therapies
American Journal of Clinical Nutrition
Nutrition Reviews
Journal of Naturopathic Medicine
Protocol Journal of Botanical Medicine

Professional Conference Tapes

Conferences of most of the medical organizations that teach nutrition and innovative medical treatments are recorded for later review or for those who were unable to attend the meetings. They are a good source of further education for professionals and interested laypeople. They may also have a catalogue of other lectures.

Audiotapes of the American College for Advancement in Medicine (ACAM) conferences from 1994 on are available from Professional

Audio Recording, telephone: 800-430-4727 or 909-593-1862; call for their catalogue of other conference tapes.

Audiotapes of ACAM conferences prior to November 1994 are available from InstaTape; telephone: 800-669-8273 or 818-303-2531. Call for their catalogue.

Audiotapes of the American Academy of Environmental Medicine conferences are available from InstaTape; telephone: 800-303-2531 or 818-303-2531.

Organizations

There are a number of organizations of health professionals that can help you locate a practitioner in your area. Starting with any of these, you should be able to find medical and nutritional support for your health needs if you have persistent problems. You may wish to start a program with a professional to help you. Some of the organizations also have members from Canada, and ACAM has many foreign members, including Canadian physicians. There are also several lay organizations doing political work and public education both in the United States and in Canada. This is a list of the most active organizations.

American College for Advancement in Medicine (ACAM)

23121 Verdugo Dr., Suite 204, Laguna Hills, CA 92653; telephone toll free: 800-532-3688 or 949-583-7666. Fax: 949-455-9679. Email: *acam@acam.org*. Web site: *www.acam.org*

For the past twenty years ACAM has been providing physician training and scientific conferences on the latest findings and emerging procedures in preventive/nutritional medicine, as well as chelation therapy for vascular disease and other degenerative disorders. ACAM's goals are to improve physician skills, knowledge, and diagnostic procedures and to develop public awareness of alternative methods of medical treatment. They publish a quarterly medical journal, the *Clinical Practice of Alternative Medicine.*

ACAM scientific conferences and physician training programs are held twice each year in different locations around the United

States. The scientific conferences are open to the public as well as professionals. The training programs now include beginning and advanced antiaging medicine, nutrition, and chelation therapy.

American Preventive Medical Association (APMA)

9912 Georgetown Pike, Suite D2, P.O. Box 458, Great Falls, VA 22066. Telephone toll free: 800-230-2762 or 703-759-0662. Fax: 703-759-6711 Web site: (*www.apma.net*)

The APMA was formed as a response to the actions of the FDA and state medical licensing boards against physicians practicing nutrition and other innovative medical treatments. It is a political action group of physicians and the public. Their mission is to achieve a health-care system in which practitioners can practice in good conscience, with the well-being of the patient foremost in their minds, and without fear of recrimination. They are constantly monitoring and taking an active role in the drafting of legislation. They were instrumental in elevating the Office of Alternative Medicine to the Center for Complementary and Alternative Medicine at the NIH (a much more effective and prestigious position).

International Society for Orthomolecular Medicine

16 Florence Ave., Toronto Ontario M2N 1E9, Canada. Telephone: 416-733-2117. Fax: 416-733-2352. Email: *centre@orthomed.org*

ISOM has been supporting orthomolecular medicine for over twenty years. They hold annual conferences to teach professionals about the latest advances in diet and nutrition as well as other innovative medical therapies. They are associated with the Canadian Schizophrenia Association, which publishes the *Journal of Orthomolecular Medicine.*

American Holistic Medical Association (AHMA)

6728 Old McLean Village Dr., McLean, VA 22101, Telephone 703-556-9745, Fax 703-556-8729. Email: *ahma@degnon.org.* Web site: (*www.holisticmedicine.org*)

The AHMA was founded in 1978 to unite fully licensed physicians who practice holistic medicine. Their mission is to support practitioners in their evolving personal and professional development and to promote an art and science that acknowledges all aspects of the individual, the family, and the planet. Holistic medicine encompasses all safe modalities of diagnosis and treatment while emphasizing the whole person.

American Academy of Environmental Medicine (AAEM)

American Financial Center, 7701 East Kellogg, Suite 625, Wichita, KS 67207–1705. Telephone: 316-684-5500. Fax: 316-684-5709. Email: *aaem@swbell.net.* Website: *www.aaem.com*

AAEM is dedicated to the purpose of education in the recognition, treatment, and prevention of illnesses induced by exposures to biologic and chemical agents encountered in air, food, and water. They have annual instructional courses in allergy and environmental medicine, clinical methods, and annual scientific meetings for physicians.

American Academy for Anti-Aging Medicine (A4M)

1510 W. Montana, Chicago, IL 60614. Telephone: 312-528-1000. Fax: 312-929-5733

A4M is a medical organization that provides information on the advances in the science of antiaging medicine that retard, stabilize, or reverse the deleterious effects of the human aging process. They hold annual scientific conferences and publish the audiotapes, videotapes and proceedings.

American Association of Naturopathic Physicians

601 Valley St., Suite 105, Seattle, WA 98109. Telephone: 206-298-0126 Fax: 206-298-0129. Web site: *www.naturopathic.org.*

Founded in 1985, the AANP is the national association representing naturopathic physicians. Naturopathic physicians are primary-health-care providers who use nontoxic therapies such as clinical nutrition, homeopathy, botanical medicine, hydrotherapy, physical medicine, and counseling. The AANP represents approximately 500 licensed naturopathic doctors.

American Chiropractic Association

1701 Clarendon Blvd., Arlington, VA 22209. Telephone: 800-986-4636. Fax: 703-243-2593. Web site: *www.amerchiro.org.*

The ACA is a professional organization representing Doctors of Chiropractic. The purpose of the ACA is to provide leadership in health care and a positive vision for the chiropractic profession and its natural approach to health and wellness.

Cancer Treatment Research Foundation

8181 S. Lewis, Tulsa, OK 74137. Telephone: 800-795-9579. Fax: 918-496-5455

They hold periodic conferences on adjuvant nutrition in the treatment and management of cancer.

Orthomolecular Health Medicine Society

2698 Pacific Ave., San Francisco, CA 94115. Telephone: 415-922-6462

This is a professional association of physicians practicing nutrition and dietary supplement therapy, as well as other innovative medical treatments. They hold annual professional conferences on nutrition and dietary supplements and other alternatives in health care.

HealthComm International

Institute for Functional Medicine, P.O. Box 1729, Gig Harbor, WA 98335. Telephone: 800-228-0622 or 253-858-4724. Fax: 253-851-9749. Web site: *www.healthcomm.com*

HealthComm International is a for-profit company that does research and holds annual conferences on functional medicine. They also have on-line education and information services.

Citizens for Health (CFH)

PO Box 2260, Boulder, CO 80306. Telephone: 800-357-2211 or 303-417-0772. FAX: 303-417-9378

Citizens for Health is a grass-roots political organization working toward freedom of choice in health care and public access to dietary supplements and information about them. They work on national and state levels and have chapters in all fifty states, Canada, and other countries.

Canadian Naturopathic Association

4174 Dundas St., Suite 303, Etobicoke, ONT M8X 1X3. Telephone: 416-233-1043. Fax: 416-233-2924. Email: *xannds@interlog.com*

Physicians and Scientists for a Healthy World (PSHW)

Dr. Ralph Idema, president. 171 Abbeyhill Drive, Kanata, ON K2L 2E9. Telephone: 613-276-8168. Fax: 613-831-4830. Email: Ralph Idema <*tropical@synapse.net*>

This Canadian organization supports dietary supplements and information about them in the Canadian Parliament and Senate to free up supplement regulations. They also have numerous other environmental interests, including lobbying the Parliament and Senate to reduce exposure to harmful chemicals such as pesticides. They support educational programs and research into environmental illness.

Appendix 3
Senate Testimony

Senate Testimony

My name is Michael Janson. I am a physician in Massachusetts with an office in Barnstable, on Cape Cod. I received my M.D. from Boston University twenty-three years ago in 1970, and then did a four-year residency in pathology. I developed an interest in nutrition, preventive medicine, and vitamin therapy after graduation and proceeded to found the Cambridge Center for Holistic Health in 1976 and more recently, the Center for Preventive Medicine, in Barnstable, Massachusetts, on Cape Cod.

I am a charter member of the American Holistic Medical Association. I am a Fellow and member of the Board of Directors of the American College for Advancement in Medicine, and the Chairman of their Scientific Advisory Committee. I am a Fellow of the International Academy of Nutrition and Preventive Medicine. I have a weekly Boston area call-in radio show reporting the latest in nutrition and preventive medicine. I am also the Vice President of the American Preventive Medical Association.

I want to thank Senator Kennedy and the members of this committee for the opportunity to clarify some of the important issues regarding dietary supplements and the FDA. I am particularly eager to relay the concerns of many of my patients and radio listeners in and around Massachusetts about their continued ability to purchase all forms of dietary supplements and to have information about their use. Many ideas relating to this form of medical care and self-care are coming out of Massachusetts. You are no doubt familiar with the reports on alternative health care by Harvard physician Dr. David Eisenberg, from the recent PBS series with Bill Moyers.

One-third of all Americans are choosing to visit alternative health-care practitioners and one-half take dietary supplements because they are willing to take personal responsibility for their own health. This costs the government nothing, and it can be clearly demonstrated that it will potentially save the government billions of dollars while enhancing the health of most Americans, with no significant risks.

The FDA has a long and clear history of bias against dietary supplements, recently evidenced by their attempted removal from the market of black currant oil capsules, claiming that it was an unsafe food additive and that the food to which it was being added was the gelatin capsule in which it was packaged. This was thrown out of court by three judges who said that the FDA was using "Alice-in-Wonderland reasoning in an effort to make an end-run around the law." FDA's own scientists and toxicologists testified that they were unaware of any safety problems with this oil. Following FDA's lead, the Texas Department of Health removed coenzyme Q_{10} from health food stores. Coenzyme Q_{10} is a remarkable, harmless substance that helps so many patients that I could hardly practice conscientiously without it. I have no doubt that it would be unavailable without passage of S. 784.

The FDA has disregarded or rejected competent scientific evidence that *Serenoa repens,* a standardized extract of the saw palmetto berry, can help shrink an enlarged prostate in middle-aged men. Meanwhile, another more expensive, more toxic, and less effective drug, for the same purpose, has been approved by the FDA. They knew that the published evidence showed the superiority of the *Serenoa,* but their action exposed 10 million men to unnecessary risks.

CSPI [Center for Science in the Public Interest] has referred to this bill as the "snake-oil promotion act." This is offensive to me and thousands of my colleagues who have clinically used supplements safely and effectively for many years. In fact, I started using them because of the vast medical literature substantiating their benefits. I have seen these benefits in seventeen years of clinical practice. I have seen almost no side effects from these products in all these years and no serious side effects. FDA-approved prescription drugs, *when used as directed,* continue to kill and injure many people annually. Dietary supplements are remarkably safe. I have been taking large amounts of them myself for many years. FDA's stated concerns about the safety of such products is not justified. Supplements are probably safer than the water that you drink to take them.

The case of L-tryptophan is important, because the FDA continues to use it as an example. It was published in both the *New England Journal of Medicine* and in the *Journal of the AMA,* in 1990, that the eosinophilia myalgia syndrome was due to a contaminant in a particular company's product. In fact, L-tryptophan has *not* been removed from the market, but only from the health food stores. It is still used in *intravenous feeding* and in *infant formulas.* The FDA has adequate safety data to permit it as an ingredient in these products.

No one wants to be the victim of fraud, and labels must be accurate. S. 784 vigorously addresses fraudulent labeling. However, *misleading labels are not as serious or dangerous a problem as the potential loss of health-enhancing dietary supplements.* But FDA's proposed regulations, which essentially ban all health claims for dietary supplements, violate the intent of the NLEA [Nutrition Labeling and Education Act]. A textbook about supplements, or scientific studies, cannot be provided by a health food store, according to FDA. Last year *The New York Times* published an article supportive of the value of dietary supplements, but a manufacturer cannot send that article, or any supportive scientific article, to its customers without concern for potential FDA regulatory action.

FDA's spokesmen mislead by carefully selecting their words when testifying before Congress in order to avoid saying what they really intend, as evidenced by their position papers. They say the debate is not about vitamins and minerals when sold in what they call reasonable potencies. What they call reasonable is far too low to be used as a guideline for optimum health. FDA considers as a drug any higher potencies of vitamins or minerals, or dietary supplements that have no essential requirement in human nutrition, or products consumed for health enhancement or therapy. *Again, the real public-health danger is from restricting access to dietary supplements, not their potential side effects.*

Specific Points

1. Without the passage of S. 784, the FDA will increase its inappropriate enforcement of misinterpreted regulations to remove a number of safe and beneficial dietary supplements from the marketplace, thus decreasing the available health choices of Americans and raising health-care costs.

2. The Dietary Supplement Health and Education Act would allow these products to remain on the market with *substantiated* health claims based on scientific data. FDA and CSPI do not speak for or protect the public on this issue, and their comments are usually unsubstantiated opinion.

3. I couldn't practice medicine responsibly without many of the substances that the FDA has already tried and will continue to try to remove from the market. I base this on what I have read from their own position papers.

4. The vast majority of the population does not want the FDA to restrict dietary supplements. To call this bill simply an industry attempt to avoid regulation belittles the enormous grass-roots movement in its favor and the intelligence of the many constituents who take and depend on dietary supplements for their continued good health.

5. The FDA blatantly misrepresents the dangers of supplements when it reports to Congress that there have been deaths from vitamin A or toxicity from essential oils, which is contrary to fact.

6. It would be ridiculous in America to have restrictions on dietary supplements but ready access to alcohol, tobacco, and "Big Macs," with all their known problems.

If I could spend a half-hour with each of you, I am convinced that you would want to take at least two or three dietary supplements that the FDA has either already tried to restrict, or will without passage of S. 784. *Serenoa* for the prostate and coenzyme Q_{10} for the heart are good examples.

In my medical practice in Massachusetts over the past seventeen years, I have seen over ten thousand patients. It is clear that many people are willing and competent to make their own choices regarding health care, including dietary supplements. They are not being duped, but they know what is at stake, and they are willing to spend their own money, not federal or state money, for the right to improve their health and prevent disease. They will not be able to continue to do this without the passage of this bill, which I strongly support.

Some of my colleagues and various researchers have also expressed similar sentiments, and I would like to report some of these to you. For example, Gladys Block, Ph.D., has made the following points:

1. The evidence of a beneficial role for [antioxidant] nutrients is extraordinarily extensive.

2. Many Americans are not consuming even minimal, let alone excessive, amounts of nutrients.

3. There is no evidence that supplement users neglect their diet or other health care—quite the contrary.

4. The evidence of benefit is increasing explosively, and conclusions formed a decade ago are insufficient to inform us.

5. FDA's role in protecting public health would be much more valuable if focused on ensuring quality of supplements and providing consumers with information.

In the reviews of the *Serenoa repens* extract studies published by the FDA in *New Developments,* of March 5, 1990, they gave their reasoning for not allowing claims for prostate improvement. Although they admitted that there was "statistically significant" improvement, they considered it not to be "clinically significant," even though it was better in all parameters than the drug that they did approve. The drug is potentially dangerous, and women who may get pregnant who are partners of men taking the drug are cautioned to avoid exposure to this partner's semen and to avoid handling the crushed tablets of the drug. It also has other side effects (impotence, decreased libido, ejaculation dysfunction). There are no known side effects from the herbal product.

The FDA does not consider only the value and safety of dietary supplements in deciding what to approve. It has other motives, including "*. . . what steps are necessary to ensure that the existence of dietary supplements on the market does not act as a disincentive for drug development.*" Also, Deputy Commissioner for Policy David Adams said that the establishment of a separate regulatory category for supplements "*. . . could undercut the exclusivity rights enjoyed by the holders of approved drug applications.*"

In a letter to *The New York Times,* September 8, 1992, Dr. Bernard Rimland said ". . . Dr. Kessler tells us that the FDA doesn't want to block the sale of vitamins. All we have to do is convince him and his fellow bureaucrats that they have been wrong for many decades in saying that vitamins are useless. Just provide the FDA with the evidence that will make them change their minds and they will let us buy all the vitamins we want. Fat chance! The FDA's stonewalling of any and all evidence favoring the use of vitamins is legendary. We could more easily convince a shark to become a vegetarian."

The evidence does not support the FDA claims that nutrients, including amino acids, are in any way a significant risk. These baseless claims mislead Congress and the public and make it dangerous to give such regulatory power to the FDA.

In case there is doubt about the regulatory intentions of the FDA, let me include some quotes from FDA officials pinpointing their position:

From the *Task Force Report on Dietary Supplements:*

". . . the task force recommends that the agency adopt a 'Dietary Supplement Limit' which would be the maximum daily intake of a given vitamin or mineral that the agency deems safe"—e.g., "the highest RDA levels listed by the National Academy of Sciences." "The Agency should take regulatory action against those supplements that exceed the above guidelines as 'unsafe food additives.' . . ."

"Amino acids should be regulated as drugs."

"If a potency is listed on the label for any nonessential substance (a dietary supplement for which there is no RDA) action would be taken against those products."

One has to question the rationale behind the FDA's proposal to redefine amino acids as "drugs." Using such an approach should suggest that sugar (sucrose) refined from beets or sugar cane, a food extraction product, should be regulated as a "drug." In fact, sugar in the American diet poses far more risks than amino acids.

Follow-up Testimony

Here is the text of what I wrote to the committee after the hearings were over, for inclusion in the official Congressional record of the hearings:

During the testimony at this hearing of Dr. David Kessler, Commissioner of the Food and Drug Administration, he made a number of misleading and false statements and a number of confusing points. I addressed some of those points in my testimony, but due to a lack of time I did not address all of them, nor did I respond adequately to reflect my concerns.

First of all on the issue of the safety of nutrients. The FDA has asked that dietary supplements meet the same standards of safety as OTC [over-the-counter] drugs. Using their own data and according to all the records of the American Association of Poison Control Centers, dietary supplements are 2,550 times safer than OTC drugs.

Dr. Kessler said that there was potential toxicity from chromium, folic acid, gamma-linolenic acid (GLA), and L-tryptophan. I am sure that he feels there is a problem with other nutrients in spite of their long record of safety based on animal and human studies and traditional use. If Dr. Kessler *feels* there is a risk, he can avoid taking these products, but only if he can *reasonably prove* a risk should the FDA be allowed to remove these from the market.

I would like to state categorically that there is no known risk from the ingestion of any of the above products at *anywhere near* the amounts that are typically used. In fact, you would probably have to take enough GLA-containing oil to get obese from the calories before it would do any other harm. No one is recommending such high doses.

Folic acid does not cause any side effects. What Dr. Kessler calls a side effect, the masking of the anemia that is an early sign of a B_{12} deficiency, is actually a therapeutic benefit. However, I recognize that a B_{12} deficiency, if prolonged, may lead to peripheral neuropathy, but this is not a side effect of the folic acid. There are now easy ways to measure B_{12} in the blood, so a physician would not have any difficulty in recognizing a deficiency. You might argue that you need to see a physician to determine this, even if people are taking folic acid on their own. However, that is moot, because a person would need a physician to recognize the anemia also. Although the dispute revolves around the dose of 400 to 1,000 *micro*grams (mcg), folic acid is safe at doses measured in *milli*grams (mg). I have seen no side effects in patients taking up to 100 mg (100,000 mcg). This dose has been used to treat gout, because, as a xanthine oxidase inhibitor, folate works like the drug allopurinol. Inhibition of xanthine oxidase may also reduce the risk of heart disease.

Chromium is a perfectly safe nutrient that can lower cholesterol and help to regulate insulin, thus improving sugar control in diabetics and hypoglycemics. Doses that I have recommended, again with no clinical or laboratory signs of toxicity, range up to 1,000 micrograms. It is safer than the drugs that are approved to lower cholesterol (e.g., lovastatin), and they have side effects such that their effect on mortality is neutral or negative.

Lovastatin actually inhibits the production of another substance, coenzyme Q_{10}, which is very important for a healthy heart, immune function, and energy production. Since coenzyme Q_{10} protects against heart disease, there is theoretical evidence, and also clinical studies, showing that this is a risk of taking the drug. And, as an aside, coenzyme Q_{10} is a substance that the Texas Department of Health, following FDA's lead, tried to remove from the health food stores in Texas.

The case of L-tryptophan deserves more comment. Dr. Kessler repeated in his testimony the claim that "they" were not sure that the eosinophilia myalgia syndrome (EMS) was due only to a contaminant. As I stated in my testimony, the *New England Journal of Medicine* and the *Journal of the AMA* both concluded that it was from a contaminant back in 1990. In the past month there have been two reports, one from the CDC by Robert Hill published in the *Archives of Environmental Contaminants and Toxicology* and one from Dr. Cluew, a professor at George Washington University, reported at a rheumatology meeting. They both concluded that the EMS was the result of a contaminant and not L-tryptophan itself.

If the FDA and Dr. Kessler do not know the older literature on the subject and they do not know the more recent literature on the subject, they are the wrong agency or the wrong personnel to be involved with the enforcement of dietary supplement regulations. There are many other reasons that I have come to this conclusion. Either we change the agency, change the personnel, or specifically limit their power with strict Congressional guidelines such as mandated in S. 784.

Dr. Kessler also revealed his true intentions inadvertently when he stated that FDA was within the law to regulate dietary supplement products that were mixtures as food additives. There is no scientific rationale for removing two safe products from the market if they happen to be mixed together, just because you have the legal authority to do so. Some products are better when they are mixed, such as GLA and vitamin E. The product lasts longer on the shelf without oxidizing because of the presence of the vitamin E. Sometimes mixtures are cheaper and sometimes they are more effective. The FDA attitude is to blow up Mount McKinley because it's there! There is no reason to expect that the FDA, with its current personnel makeup and level of authority, will suddenly start to treat dietary supplements more equitably than they have for decades.

Dr. Kessler left the impression that all the bottles of products that he displayed, in his grandstanding gesture, were labeled with false claims. He presented only one that had a false claim on the label. (No one at the hearing actually examined the label, but I have no doubt that there are occasional false claims, which generally are not a great risk to the public health.) Most of those products were properly labeled, but FDA agents were able to cajole someone at a health food store to suggest to them that the product would be useful for a specific health problem. The manufacturers or distributors are inappropriately being held liable for the actions of retail clerks. If a clerk in a market said to take prunes for constipation, that would be an unsubstantiated health claim according to the FDA, and they could have put a box of prunes on the table with all those bottles.

When confronted with the toxicity of FDA-approved drugs, which kill so many people annually, Dr. Kessler replied with his "canned" comment that "half of our drugs are derived from plants." This is a clear misrepresentation and designed to mislead. Many pharmaceuticals are plant extracts that have been significantly altered so that they can be patented, and this alteration usually increases their toxicity. Also, many of them are synthetic analogs of plant products, not the plants themselves. You might as well say that they are made from carbon, nitrogen and oxygen, which we encounter every day! Further, many of the most widely used and most expensive drugs are totally synthetic and have nothing to do with plants. Antiulcer drugs, anti-inflammatory drugs, antianxiety drugs, newer cardiac drugs, and antihypertensives are not plant products. They cost many Americans lots of money and have numerous side effects. They are necessary for many patients but are widely overused. This is partly because physicians have no access, in the normal course of their work, to the information about dietary supplements that should be disseminated widely. This would lessen the need for drugs and enhance the health of all Americans, while reducing the medical-care crisis that we are now facing.

Dr. Kessler decried the variety of health claims being made for evening primrose oil. He is perhaps unaware of the hundreds of studies in the literature supporting most of those uses. It is not surprising that a physician would be skeptical of something that seems to help so many illnesses. But it is a mistake to be blinded by skepticism from seeing the scientific evidence. Because GLA [from evening primrose and other oils] is a precursor to regulatory substances known as "prostaglandins," it has wide-ranging metabolic effects. It does help to lower blood pressure, reduce or cure atopic dermatitis, relieve PMS, reduce cholesterol and inflammation, and help asthmatics and allergic patients. These are the many effects of the prostaglandins that are made from this important fatty acid. It is therefore not "incredible" to someone who bothers to look up the scientific documentation and who understands the metabolic rationale.

I want to reaffirm that these claims were *not* on the labels of these products, but they *are* in the medical literature. Also, I have observed in my practice the above-stated clinical effects, and have reviewed many of the studies substantiating some of the claims that the FDA agents heard from health food store clerks. The FDA should be doing everything in its power to disseminate this information and encouraging manufacturers to disseminate it also, as long as it is in the medical literature and not misleading. Instead, they are an obstacle to information exchange and are themselves misleading. This can only be changed if the FDA stops confusing its role of regulating real danger and fraud with the role of being the arbiter and promoter of truth as they see it. Passage of S. 784 will ensure a more sane approach to regulation, availability of dietary supplements, and truthful health claims.

When Dr. Kessler says that they "plan to take no products off the market," that is a dramatic shift from what they have proposed in all their written material until now. With such waffling, confusion, and misleading testimony, the FDA cannot be expected to take an honest and human approach to regulating such an important component of our health care.

I have read Dr. Linus Pauling's letter addressed to the committee supporting the Dietary Supplements Act. I hope it is included in the record because it is an eloquent statement that combines common sense, science, reason, and compassion.

Linus Pauling's Testimony

Linus Pauling, the only person ever to have won two unshared Nobel prizes, died in 1994 at the age of ninety-three. He pursued his research and directed the Linus Pauling Institute of Science and Medicine until shortly before his death from prostate cancer. He partially credited his long life (his parents had both died quite young) to his large doses of vitamin C (18 g per day) and other dietary supplements.

Here is the text of Linus Pauling's letter to the Senate committee, reprinted with permission of his family:

I am deeply concerned with the current state of affairs revolving around the issue of dietary supplements and related substances. The overwhelming body of evidence in the official medical and scientific indices regarding the efficacy and safety of vitamins, minerals, enzymes, amino acids, herbs, and other nutritionally related substances is obviously being ignored or, at best, misinterpreted to suit the special interests of a medical and political contingency. The volumes of respected historical data and conclusive current research in regard to these substances and their value in healthcare far outweigh single isolated instances of contamination, not to mention clinically and statistically unsubstantiated claims of toxicity. The manipulation of empirical credibility by political or economic egos is not to be tolerated or exonerated.

As a scientist, chemist, physicist, crystallographer, molecular biologist, and medical researcher, I have spent a lifetime in pursuit of expert knowledge. This issue involving the definition, regulation, and censorship of dietary supplements and associated information goes far beyond this hearing. It touches upon the very fiber of our human and constitutional rights. It mandates monopolization of the healthcare industry by creating an economic premise that will eventually eliminate those unable to meet its unrealistic requirements. These demands would require millions of dollars in research and excessive time constraints to prove the safety of substances already historically and statistically within considerable safety margins.

In the scientific and medical communities, among those of reputable and significant knowledge, the votes have already been cast in favor of nontoxic therapies that are effective and affordable. This issue of agency determination of definitions and regulations overrides the individual's freedom of choice in healthcare, and inhibits free access to vitamin information that better enables a person to make an informed intelligent decision regarding services that could be of significant value in the prevention and treatment of disease, making it mandatory that they be made available only as "drugs," and under the jurisdiction therefore of the medical community. This ultimately enslaves a population to becoming chemically, psychologically, and economically dependent, rather than being actively responsible for its own well being. Billions of dollars and millions of lives are at risk of being jeopardized in this ruthless campaign to subjugate the health industry to being puppets of a legislated system of lobbying efforts.

It is imperative to maintain the highest quality of purity, safety, and performance in regard to consumer products and services. However, the subversive actions of raids at gunpoint, confiscation of patients' records and personal property, and warrantless censorship and banning of information and substances that are statistically proven to be of benefit are blatant violations of human and constitutional rights. As a scientist, I am appalled at the audacity of those challenging these rights; as a citizen, I am compelled to voice my indignation at being considered incapable of being in charge of my own health. The medical community needs to become a partner, not a dictator, in the healthcare system.

Over a quarter of a century ago, I became interested in nutrient compounds and their effects on human health. The old professors of nutrition who helped to develop the science of nutrition seemed complacent with their accomplishments and ignored the new discoveries that were being made in medicine, biochemistry, and molecular biology. They continued to teach their students the old ideas, many of them incomplete or incorrect, resulting in principles and practices that have denied the public proper access to new concepts and therapies.

Physicians themselves, though dedicated and intelligent, are virtually untrained in the area of nutritional science and metabolic therapy, other than conventional drug modalities and allopathic procedures. If there is to be a concerted effort to regulate and eliminate toxic substances, it would serve the issue far better to address the abuse of drugs and treatment procedures that are the cause of hundreds of thousands of medical catastrophies and deaths per year, which could possibly be avoided by improving medical education of the physicians and the public as to nutritional alternatives in healthcare maintenance.

At this hearing, I urge you to consider seriously the ramifications of crippling the full disclosure of information to the public regarding health research, and the unnecessary regulations and improper definitions of dietary supplements as drugs. This implies a direct infringement of medical freedom of choice and the First Amendment, freedom of speech, allowing for a dangerous precedent of censorship that could generate epidemic problems not only in human health but human values. The Constitution of the World Health Organization, as mandated in conformity with the Charter of the United Nations, of which the United States is a signatory, states:

"Health is a state of complete physical, mental and social well-being and not merely the absence of disease or infirmity. The enjoyment of the highest standard of health is one of the fundamental rights of every human being without distinction of race, religion, political belief, economic or social condition. The health of all peoples is fundamental to the attainment of peace and security and is dependent upon the fullest cooperation of individuals and states. The extension to all peoples of the benefits of medical, psychological and related knowledge is essential to the fullest attainment of health. Informed opinion and active cooperation on the part of the public are of the utmost importance in the improvement of the health of the people." (Geneva, 1976)

This hearing is paramount to the determination of the Dietary Supplements Act, S-784. I submit to you the history-making moment that we are facing. As representatives of the people, consider not only the medical and scientific implications, but the humanity of your decisions. We are on the threshold of a new paradigm. The future of our self-determination as humankind depends upon our right to life and to live in freedom. Herophiles in 300 B.C. stated: "When Health is absent, Wisdom cannot reveal itself, Art cannot become manifest, Strength cannot be exerted, Wealth is useless, and Reason is powerless."

I trust that your reason will surpass the rhetoric, and that your wisdom will reveal the truth in support of the Dietary Supplements Act.

Sincerely,

Linus Pauling

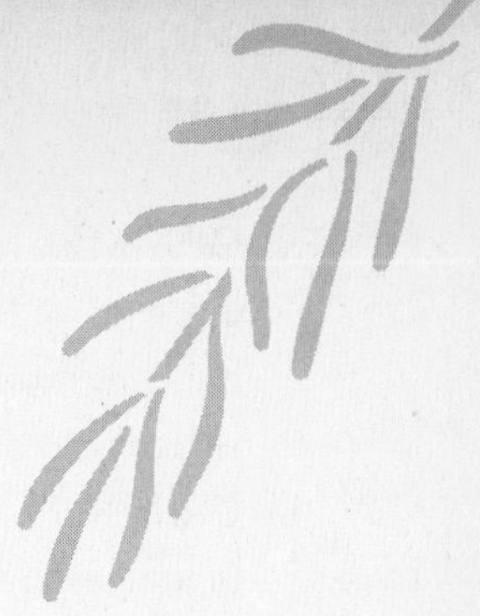

Selected References

References have been chosen to represent the science behind the information in the text.

Chapter 1. Why You Need Vitamins

1. Lamm, D. L., Riggs, D. R., Shriver, J. S., van Gilder, P. F., Rach, J. F., DeHaven, J. I. Megadose vitamins in bladder cancer: a double-blind clinical trial. *J Urol* 1994 Jan; 151(1):21–26.
2. Jaakkola, K., Lahteenmaki, P., Laakso, J., Harju, E., Tykka, H., Mahlberg, K. Treatment with antioxidant and other nutrients in combination with chemotherapy and irradiation in patients with small-cell lung cancer. *Anticancer Res* 1992 May–Jun; 12(3):599–606.
3. Riggs, D. R., DeHaven, J. I., Lamm, D. L. Allium sativum (garlic) treatment for murine transitional cell carcinoma. *Cancer* 1997 May 15; 79(10):1987–94.
4. Patterson, R. E., White, E., Kristal, A. R., Neuhouser, M. L., Potter, J.D. Vitamin supplements and cancer risk: the epidemiologic evidence. *Cancer Causes Control* 1997 Sep; 8(5):786–802.

5. Gey, K. F., Stahelin, H. B., Eichholzer, M. Poor plasma status of carotene and vitamin C is associated with higher mortality from ischemic heart disease and stroke: Basel Prospective Study. *Clin Investig* 1993 Jan; 71(1):3–6.
6. Odeh, R. M., Cornish, L. A. Natural antioxidants for the prevention of atherosclerosis. *Pharmacotherapy* 1995 Sep–Oct; 15(5):648–59.
7. Quillin, P. Adjuvant Nutrition in Cancer Treatment. *J Advancement Med,* Fall 1995; 8(3):177–91.
8. Steinberg, D. Antioxidant vitamins and coronary heart disease. *New Engl J Med* 328(20):1487–89, May 20, 1993.
9. Taylor, A. Associations between nutrition and cataract. *Nutr Rev* 47:225, 1989.
10. Levine, G. N., Frei, B., Koulouris, S. N., Gerhard, M.D., Keaney, J. F., Vita, J. Ascorbic acid reverses endothelial vasomotor dysfunction in patients with coronary artery disease. *Circulation* 93(6):1107–13, March 15, 1996.
11. Shklar, G., Schwartz, J., Trickler, D., Reid, S. Regression of experimental cancer by oral administration of combined alpha-tocopherol and beta-carotene. *Nutr Cancer* 12:321–25, 1989.
12. Malter, M., Schriever, G., Eilber U. Natural killer cells, vitamins, and other blood components of vegetarian and omnivorous men. *Nutr Cancer* 1989; 12(3):271–78.
13. Butland, B. K. Heart disease in British vegetarians. *Am J Clin Nutr* 1988 Sep; 48(3 Suppl):830–32.
14. Frentzel-Beyme, R., Claude, J., Eilber, U. Mortality among German vegetarians: first results after five years of follow-up. *Nutr Cancer* 1988; 11(2):117–26.
15. Hu, F. B., Stampfer, M. J., Manson, J. E., et al. Dietary fat intake and the risk of coronary heart disease in women. *N Engl J Med* 1997; 337:1491–99.
16. Gjonca, A., Bobak, M. Long life expectancy linked to Albanian diet. *Lancet* 1997; 350:1815–17.
17. Bijnen, F. C. H., Caspersen, C. J., Feskens, E. J. M. Physical activity and 10-year mortality from cardiovascular diseases and all causes. *Arch Intern Med.* 1998; 158:1499–1505.

Chapter 2. "Orthomolecular" Medicine: The Right Molecules in the Right Amounts

1. Hoffer, A., Osmond, H., Callbeck, M. J., Kahan, I. Treatment of schizophrenia with nicotinic acid and nicotinamide. *J Clin Exper Psychopathol* 18:131–58, 1957.
2. Osmond, H., Hoffer, A. Schizophrenia: A new approach III. *J Ment Sci* 105:653–73. 1959.
3. Osmond, H., Hoffer, A. Massive niacin treatment in schizophrenia: Review of a nine-year study. *Lancet* 1:316–20, 1962.
4. Pauling, L. Orthomolecular psychiatry. Varying the concentrations of substances normally present in the human body may control mental disease. *Science* 1968 Apr; 160(825):265–71.
5. ———. Proceedings: On the molecular environment of the mind: orthomolecular theory. *Psychopharmacol Bull.* 1974 Oct; 10(4): 6–7.
6. Cameron, E., Pauling, L. The orthomolecular treatment of cancer. I. The role of ascorbic acid in host resistance. *Chem Biol Interact.* 1974 Oct; 9(4):273–83.
7. Lazarou, J., Pomeranz, B. H., Corey, P. N. Incidence of adverse drug reactions in hospitalized patients: a meta-analysis of prospective studies. *JAMA* 1998 Apr 15; 279(15):1200–5.
8. *Mental and Elemental Nutrients,* Carl Pfeiffer, M.D., Ph.D.
9. Levine, M. New concepts in the biology and biochemistry of ascorbic acid. *N Engl J Med* 1986 Apr 3; 314(14):892–902.

Chapter 3. Fat-Soluble Nutrients

1. Gerster, H. Vitamin A—functions, dietary requirements and safety in humans. *Int J Vitam Nutr Res* 1997; 67(2):71–90.
2. Ross, A. C., and Stephensen, C. B. Vitamin A and retinoids in antiviral responses. *FASEB J* 1996 Jul; 10(9):979–85.
3. Garewal, H. S., Meyskens, F. L., Killen, D., et al. Response of oral leukoplakia to beta-carotene. *J Clin Oncol* 8:1715, 1990.
4. Shklar, G., Schwartz, J., Trickler, D., Reid, S. Regression of experimental cancer by oral administration of combined alpha-tocopherol and beta-carotene. *Nutr Cancer* 12:321–25, 1989.

5. Santos, M., Meydani, S. N., Leka, L., et al. Elderly male natural killer cell activity is enhanced by beta-carotene supplementation. *FASEB J* 9:A436, 1995.
6. Watson, R. R., Prabhala, R. H., Plezia, P. M., Alberts D. S. Effect of beta-carotene on lymphocyte subpopulations in elderly humans: evidence for a dose-response relationship. *Am J Clin Nut* 53:90, 1991.
7. Yeum, K. J., Taylor, A., Tang, G., Russell, R. M. Measurement of carotenoids, retinoids, and tocopherols in human lenses. *Invest Ophthalmol Vis Sci* 1995 Dec; 36(13):2756–61.
8. Giovannucci, E., Ascherio, A., Rimm, E. B., Stampfer, M. J., Colditz, G. A., Willett, W. C. Intake of carotenoids and retinol in relation to risk of prostate cancer. *J Natl Cancer Inst* 1995 Dec 6; 87(23):1767–76.
9. Le Marchand, L., Hankin, J. H., Bach, F., et al. An ecological study of diet and lung cancer in the South Pacific. *Int J Cancer* 1995 Sep 27; 63(1):18–23.
10. Snodderly, D. M. Evidence for protection against age-related macular degeneration by carotenoids and antioxidant vitamins. *Am J Clin Nutr* 1995 Dec; 62(6 Suppl):1448S–61S.
11. Alpha-Tocopherol, Beta-carotene Cancer Prevention Study Group, The effect of vitamin E and beta-carotene on the incidence of lung cancer and other cancers in male smokers. *N Engl J Med* 330:1029–35, 1994.
12. Omenn, G. S., Goodman, G., Thornquist, M., Grizzle, J., Rosenstock, L., Barnhart, S., et al. The beta-carotene and retinol efficacy trial (CARET) for chemoprevention of lung cancer in high risk populations: smokers and asbestos-exposed workers. *Cancer Res* 1; 54(7 Suppl):2038s-2043s, Apr, 1994.
13. Gey, K. F. Inverse correlation of vitamin E and ischemic heart disease. *Int J Vitam Nutr Res Suppl* 1989; 30:224–31.
14. Gey, K. F., Stahelin, H. B., Puska, P., Evans, A. Relationship of plasma level of vitamin C to mortality from ischemic heart disease. *Ann N Y Acad Sci* 1987; 498:110–23.
15. Steinberg, D. Antioxidants and atherosclerosis, a current assessment. Circulation 84(3):1420–25, September 1991.

16. Steinberg, D. Antioxidant vitamins and coronary heart disease. *New Engl J Med* 1993 May 20; 328(20):1487–89.
17. Gaziano, J. M. Antioxidant vitamins and coronary artery disease risk. *Am J Med* 1994 Sep 26; 97(3A):18S–21S.
18. Rimm, E. B., Stampfer, M. J., Ascherio, A., Giovannucci, E., Colditz, G. A., Willett, W. C. Vitamin E consumption and the risk of coronary heart disease in men. *N Engl J Med* 1993 May 20; 328(20):1450–56.
19. Steiner, M. Influence of vitamin E on platelet function in humans. *J Am Coll Nutr* 9(5): 554, 1990.
20. Meydani, S., Barkland, M. P., Liu, S., et al. Vitamin E supplementation enhances cell-mediated immunity in healthy elderly subjects. *Am J Clin Nutr* 52: 557–63, 1990.
21. Nalbandian, R. M., Henry, R. L. A proposed comprehensive pathophysiology of thrombotic thrombocytopenic purpura with implicit novel tests and therapies. *Seminars in Thrombosis and Hemostasis* 6:356, 1980.
22. Gilbert, V. A., Zebrowski, E. J., Chan, A. C. Differential effect of megavitamin E on prostacycline and thromboxane synthesis in streptozatocin-induced diabetic rats. *Horm Metab Res* 15:320, 1983.
23. Taylor, A. Associations between nutrition and cataract. *Nutr Rev* 47:225, 1989.
24. Robertson, J. M. C. D., Donner, A. P., Trevithick, J. R. Vitamin E intake and risk of cataracts in humans. *Ann N Y Acad Sci* 570:372–82, 1989.
25. Tutuncu, N. B., Bayraktar, M., Varli, K. Reversal of defective nerve conduction with vitamin E supplementation in type 2 diabetes: a preliminary study. *Diabetes Care* 1998 Nov; 21(11):1915–18.
26. Thomas, M. K., Lloyd-Jones, D. M., Thadhani, R. I., et al. Hypovitaminosis D in medical patients. *N Engl J Med* 1998 Mar 19; 338(12):777–83.
27. Jacques, P. F., Felson, D. T., Tucker, K. L., Mahnken, B., et al. Plasma 25-hydroxyvitamin D and its determinants in an elderly population sample. *Am J Clin Nutr* 1997 Oct; 66(4):929–36.

28. Craciun, A. M., Wolf, J., Knapen, M. H., Brouns, F., Vermeer, C. Improved bone metabolism in female elite athletes after vitamin K supplementation. *Int J Sports Med* 1998 Oct; 19(7):479–84.
29. Mijares, M. E., Nagy, E., Guerrero, B., Arocha-Pinango, C. L. Vitamin K: biochemistry, function, and deficiency. *Review. Invest Clin* 1998 Sep; 39(3):213–29.

Chapter 4. *Water-Soluble Nutrients*

1. Head, K. A. Ascorbic acid in the prevention and treatment of cancer. *Altern Med Rev* 1998 Jun; 3(3):174–86.
2. Tomoda, H., Yoshitake, M., Morimoto, K., Aoki, N. Possible prevention of postangioplasty restenosis by ascorbic acid. *Am J Cardiol* 1996 Dec 1; 78(11):1284–6.
3. Bassenge, E., Fink, N., Skatchkov, M., Fink, B. Dietary supplement with vitamin C prevents nitrate tolerance. *J Clin Invest* 1998 Jul 1; 102(1):67–71.
4. Cohen, H. A., Neuman, I., Nahum, H. Blocking effect of vitamin C in exercise-induced asthma. *Arch Pediatr Adolesc Med.* 1997; 151:367–70.
5. Bielory, L., and Gandhi, R. Asthma and vitamin C. *Ann Allerg* 1994; 73:89–96.
6. Pandey, D. K., Shekelle, R., Selwyn, B. J., Tangney, C., Stamler, J. Dietary vitamin C and beta-carotene and risk of death in middle-aged men. The Western Electric Study. *Am J Epidemiol* 1995 Dec 15; 142(12):1269–78.
7. Gale, C. R., Martyn, C. N., Winter, P. D., Cooper, C. Vitamin C and risk of death from stroke and coronary heart disease in cohort of elderly people. *BMJ* 1995 Jun 17; 310(6994):1563–66.
8. Todd, S., Woodward, M., Bolton-Smith, C. An investigation of the relationship between antioxidant vitamin intake and coronary heart disease in men and women using logistic regression analysis. *J Clin Epidemiol* 1995 Feb; 48(2):307–16.
9. Vita, J. A., Keaney, J. F., Jr., Raby, K. E., et al. Low plasma ascorbic acid independently predicts the presence of an unstable coronary syndrome. *J Am Coll Cardiol* 1998 Apr; 31(5):980–86.

10. Watanabe, H., et al. Vitamin C and nitrate tolerance. *J Am Coll Cardiol* 1998; 31:1323–29.
11. Ness, A. R., Khaw, K. T., Bingham, S., Day, N. E. Vitamin C status and blood pressure. *J Hypertens* 1996 Apr; 14(4):503–8.
12. Bucca, C., Rolla, G., Oliva, A., Farina, J. C. Effect of vitamin C on histamine bronchial responsiveness of patients with allergic rhinitis. *Ann Allergy* 65: 311–14, October 1990.
13. Podoshin, L., Gertner, R., Fradis, M. Treatment of perennial allergic rhinitis with ascorbic acid solution [letter]. *Ear Nose Throat J* 70(1): 54–55, January 1991.
14. Clemetson, C. A. B. Histamine and ascorbic acid in human blood. *J Nutr* 110(4): 662–68, April 1980.
15. Pauling, L. *Vitamin C and the Common Cold,* San Francisco: W.H. Freeman & Co, 1970.
16. Pauling, L. *Vitamin C, the Common Cold and the Flu,* San Francisco: W.H. Freeman & Co, 1976.
17. Anderson, T. W., Reid, D. B., Beaton, G. H. Vitamin C and the common cold: a double-blind trial. *Canad Med Assoc J* 107:503, 1972.
18. Ritzel, G. Critical evaluation of vitamin C as a prophylactic and therapeutic agent in colds. *Helvetica Med Acta* 28:63, 1961.
19. Hume, R., and Weyers, E. Changes in leucocyte ascorbic acid during the common cold. *Scottish Med J* 18:3–7, 1973.
20. Lehr, H. A., Frei, B., Olofsson, A. M., Carew, T. E., Arfors, K. E. Protection from oxidized LDL-induced leukocyte adhesion to microvascular and macrovascular endothelium in vivo by vitamin C but not by vitamin E. *Circulation* 91(5):1525–32, March 1995.
21. Retsky, K. L., Freeman, M. W., Frei, B. Ascorbic acid oxidation products protect human low density lipoprotein against atherogenic modification—anti- rather than pro-oxidant activity of vitamin C in the presence of transition metals. *J Biol Chem,* 1993 January 268(2): 1304–09.
22. Levine, G. N., Frei, B., Koulouris, S. N., Gerhard, M. D., Keaney, J. F., Vita, J. Ascorbic acid reverses endothelial vasomotor dysfunction in patients with coronary artery disease. *Circulation* 1996 March 15 93(6):1107–13.

23. Heitzer, T., Just, H., Munzel, T. Antioxidant vitamin C improves endothelial dysfunction in smokers. *Circulation* 1996 July 1 94(1):6–9.
24. Frei, B. Does vitamin C cause genetic damage? *Linus Pauling Institute Newsletter* 1998 Fall/Winter, pp. 4–5.
25. Mattimoe, D., and Newton, W. High-dose riboflavin for migraine prophylaxis. *J Fam Pract* 1998 Jul; 47(1):11.
26. Schoenen, J., Jacquy, J., Lenaerts, M. Effectiveness of high-dose riboflavin in migraine prophylaxis. A randomized controlled trial. *Neurology* 1998 Feb; 50(2):466–70.
27. Hoffer, A., Osmond, H., Callbeck, M. J., Kahan, I. Treatment of schizophrenia with nicotinic acid and nicotinamide. *J Clin Exper Psychopathol* 1957 18:131–58.
28. Osmond, H., and Hoffer, A. Massive niacin treatment in schizophrenia: Review of a nine-year study. *Lancet* 1962 1:316–20.
29. Capuzzi, D. M., Guyton, J. R., Morgan, J. M., et al. Efficacy and safety of an extended-release niacin (Niaspan): a long-term study. *Am J Cardiol* 1998 Dec 17; 82(12A):74U–81U; discussion 85U–86U.
30. Guyton, J. R. Effect of niacin on atherosclerotic cardiovascular disease. *Am J Cardiol* 1998 Dec 17; 82(12A):18U–23U.
31. O'Hara, J., Jolly, P. N., Nicol, C. G. The therapeutic efficacy of inositol nicotinate (Hexopal) in intermittent claudication: a controlled trial. *Br J Clin Pract* 1988 Sep; 42(9):377–83.
32. Sunderland, G. T., Belch, J. J., Sturrock, R. D., Forbes, C. D., McKay, A. J. A double blind randomised placebo controlled trial of hexopal in primary Raynaud's disease. *Clin Rheumatol* 1988 Mar; 7(1):46–49.
33. Vorberg, G. Effective therapy of chronic arterial circulatory disorders with Nico-Padutin forte. *MMW Munch Med Wochenschr* 1976 Oct 29; 118(44):1429–32.
34. Borets, V. M., Lis, M. A., Pyrochkin, V. M., et al. Therapeutic efficacy of pantothenic acid preparations in ischemic heart disease patients. *Vopr Pitan* 1987 Mar-Apr; (2):15–17.
35. Arsenio, L., Caronna, S., Lateana, M., et al. Hyperlipidemia, diabetes and atherosclerosis: efficacy of treatment with pantethine. *Acta Biomed Ateneo Parmense* 1984; 55:25–42.

36. Gaddi, A., Descovich, G. C., Noseda, G., et al. Controlled evaluation of pantethine, a natural hypolipidemic compound, in patients with different forms of hyperlipoproteinemia. *Atherosclerosis* 1984; 50:73–83.
37. Donati, C., Bertieri, R. S., Barbi, G. Pantethine, diabetes mellitus and atherosclerosis. Clinical study of 1045 patients. *Clin Ter* 1989; 128:411–22.
38. Aybak, M., Sermet, A., Ayyildiz, M. O., Karakilcik, A. Z. Effect of oral pyridoxine hydrochloride supplementation on arterial blood pressure in patients with essential hypertension. *Arzneimittelforschung* 1995 Dec; 45(12):1271–73.
39. Selhub, J., Jacques, P. F., Wilson, P. W., Rush, D., Rosenberg, I. H. Vitamin status and intake as primary determinants of homocysteinemia in an elderly population. *JAMA* 1993 Dec 8; 270(22):2693–98.
40. Ellis, J. M., and McCully, K. S. Prevention of myocardial infarction by vitamin B6. *Res Commun Mol Pathol Pharmacol* 1995 Aug; 89(2):208–20.
41. Lal, K. J., Dakshinamurti, K., Thliveris, J. The effect of vitamin B_6 on the systolic blood pressure of rats in various animal models of hypertension. *J Hypertens* 1996 Mar; 14(3):355–63.
42. Bernstein, A. L., and Dinesen, J. S. Brief communication: effect of pharmacologic doses of vitamin B_6 on carpal tunnel syndrome, electroencephalographic results, and pain. *J Am Coll Nutr* 1993 Feb; 12(1):73–76.
43. Ellis, J. M., Folkers, K., et al. A deficiency of vitamin B_6 is a plausible molecular basis of the retinopathy of patients with diabetes mellitus. *Biochem Biophys Res Commun* 1991 Aug 30; 179(1):615–19.
44. Abbas, Z. G., and Swai, A. B. Evaluation of the efficacy of thiamine and pyridoxine in the treatment of symptomatic diabetic peripheral neuropathy. *East Afr Med J* 1997 Dec; 74(12):803–8.
45. Schaumburg, H., Kaplan, J., Windebank, A., et al. Sensory neuropathy from pyridoxine abuse. A new megavitamin syndrome. *N Engl J Med* 1983 Aug 25; 309(8):445–48.
46. Locksmith, G. J., and Duff, P. Preventing neural tube defects: the importance of periconceptional folic acid. *Obstet Gynecol* 1998 Jun; 91(6):1027–34.

47. Mason, J. B., and Levesque, T. Folate: effects on carcinogenesis and the potential for cancer chemoprevention. *Oncology* (Huntingt) 1996 Nov; 10(11):1727–36, 1742–43; discussion 1743–44.
48. Butterworth, C. E., Jr., Hatch, K. D., Gore, H., Mueller, H., Krumdieck, C. L. Improvement in cervical dysplasia associated with folic acid therapy in users of oral contraceptives. *Am J Clin Nutr* 1982 Jan; 35(1):73–82.
49. VanEenwyk, J., Davis, F. G., Colman, N. Folate, vitamin C, and cervical intraepithelial neoplasia. *Cancer Epidemiol Biomarkers Prev* 1992 Jan–Feb; 1(2):119–24.
50. Butterworth, C. E., Jr. Effect of folate on cervical cancer. Synergism among risk factors. *Ann N Y Acad Sci* 1992 Sep 30; 669:293–99.
51. Flynn, M. A., Irvin, W., Krause, G. The effect of folate and cobalamin on osteoarthritic hands. *J Am Coll Nutr* 1994 Aug; 13(4):351–6.
52. Lewis, A. S., Murphy, L., McCalla, C. Fleary, M., Purcell, S. Inhibition of mammalian xanthine oxidase by folate compounds and amethopterin. *J Biol Chem* 1984 Jan 10; 259:12–15.
53. Spector, T., and Ferone, R. Folic acid does not inactivate xanthine oxidase. *J Biol Chem* 1984 Sep 10; 259(17):10784–86.

Chapter 5. *Mineral Supplements*

1. Laskey, M. A., et al. Bone changes after 3 mo of lactation: influence of calcium intake, breast-milk output, and vitamin D–receptor genotype. *Am J Clin Nutr* 1998 Apr; 67(4):685–92.
2. Bostick, R. M., Kushi, L. H., Wu, Y. Relation of calcium, vitamin D, and dairy food intake to ischemic heart disease mortality among postmenopausal women. *Am J Epidemiol* 1999 Jan 15; 149(2):151–61.
3. Hosking, D. J., Ross, P. D., Thompson, D. E., et al. Evidence that increased calcium intake does not prevent early postmenopausal bone loss. *Clin Ther* 1998 Sep–Oct; 20(5):933–44.
4. Lau, E. M., Kwok, T., Woo, J., Ho, S. C. Bone mineral density in Chinese elderly female vegetarians, vegans, lacto-vegetarians and omnivores. *Eur J Clin Nutr* 1998 Jan; 52(1):60–4.

5. Baron, J. A., Beach, M., Mandel, J. S., et al. Calcium supplements for the prevention of colorectal adenomas. Calcium Polyp Prevention Study Group. *N Engl J Med* 1999 Jan 14; 340(2):101–7.
6. Pak, C. Y. Calcium metabolism. *J Am Coll Nutr* 1989; 8 Suppl:46S–53S.
7. White, J. E. Osteoporosis: strategies for prevention. *Nurse Pract* 1986 Sep; 11(9):36–46, 50.
8. Walker, A. F., De Souza, M. C., Vickers, M. F., et al. Magnesium supplementation alleviates premenstrual symptoms of fluid retention. *J Womens Health* 1998 Nov; 7(9):1157–65.
9. Nattel, S., Turmel, N., Macleod, R., Solymoss, B. C. Actions of intravenous magnesium on ventricular arrhythmias caused by acute myocardial infarction. *J Pharmacol Exp Ther* 1991 Nov; 259(2):939–46.
10. Woods, K. L., Fletcher, S., Roffe, C., Haider, Y. Intravenous magnesium sulphate in suspected acute myocardial infarction: results of the second Leicester Intravenous Magnesium Intervention Trial (LIMIT-2) *Lancet* 1992 Jun 27; 339(8809):1553–58.
11. Keren, A., Tzivoni, D. Magnesium therapy in ventricular arrhythmias. *Pacing Clin Electrophysiol* 1990 Jul; 13(7):937–45.
12. Dyckner, T., Wester, P. O., Widman, L. Effects of peroral magnesium on plasma and skeletal muscle electrolytes in patients on long-term diuretic therapy. *Int J Cardiol* 1988 Apr; 19(1):81–87.
13. Spatling, L., Spatling, G. Magnesium supplementation in pregnancy.A double-blind study. *Br J Obstet Gynaecol* 1988 Feb; 95(2):120–25.
14. Chouinard, G., Beauclair, L., Geiser, R., Etienne, P. A pilot study of magnesium aspartate hydrochloride (Magnesiocard) as a mood stabilizer for rapid cycling bipolar affective disorder patients. *Prog Neuropsychopharmacol Biol Psychiatry* 1990; 14(2):171–80.
15. Sebekova, K., Revusova, V., Polakovicova, D., Drahosova, J., Zverkova, D., Dzurik, R. Anti-hypertensive treatment with magnesium-aspartate-dichloride and its influence on peripheral serotonin metabolism in man: a subacute study. *Cor Vasa* 1992; 34(5–6):390–401.
16. Witteman, J. C., Grobbee, D. E., Derkx, F. H., Bouillon R., de Bruijn A. M., Hofman A. Reduction of blood pressure with oral magnesium

supplementation in women with mild to moderate hypertension. *Am J Clin Nutr* 1994 Jul; 60(1):129–35.

17. Heinritzi, K., Ehrenberg, A., Berner, H. Prevention of myopathies and cardiomyopathies in swine using magnesium aspartate hydrochloride. *Berl Munch Tierarztl Wochenschr* 1993 Jul; 106(7):224–27.
18. Attias, J., Weisz, G., Almog, S., et al. Oral magnesium intake reduces permanent hearing loss induced by noise exposure. *Am J Otolaryngol* 1994 Jan–Feb; 15(1):26–32.
19. Sempertegui, F., Estrella, B., Correa, E., et al. Effects of short-term zinc supplementation on cellular immunity, respiratory symptoms, and growth of malnourished Equadorian children. *Eur J Clin Nutr* 1996 Jan; 50(1):42–46.
20. Goetzl, E. J., Banda, M. J., Leppert, D. Matrix metalloproteinases in immunity. *J Immunol* 1996 Jan 1; 156(1):1–4.
21. Kodama, H. Essential trace elements and immunity. *Nippon Rinsho* 1996 Jan; 54(1):46–51.
22. Saha, A. R., Hadden, E. M., Hadden, J. W. Zinc induces thymulin secretion from human thymic epithelial cells in vitro and augments splenocyte and thymocyte responses in vivo. *Int J Immunopharmacol* 1995 Sep; 17(9):729–33.
23. Mocchegiani, E., Santarelli, L., Muzzioli, M., Fabris, N. Reversibility of the thymic involution and of age-related peripheral immune dysfunctions by zinc supplementation in old mice. *Int J Immunopharmacol* 1995 Sep; 17(9):703–18.
24. Prasad, A. S. Zinc: an overview. *Nutrition* 1995 Jan–Feb; 11(1 Suppl):93–99.
25. Maganto, P. E. Zinc in prostatic physiopathology. I. Role of zinc in the physiology and biochemistry of the prostatic gland. *Arch Esp Urol* 1979 Mar–Apr; 32(2):143–52.
26. Leake, A., Chisholm, G. D., Habib, F. K. The effect of zinc on the 5 alpha-reduction of testosterone by the hyperplastic human prostate gland. *J Steroid Biochem* 1984 Feb; 20(2):651–55.
27. Merluzzi, V. J., Cipriano, D., McNeil, D., et al. Evaluation of zinc complexes on the replication of rhinovirus 2 in vitro. *Res Commun Chem Pathol Pharmacol* 1989 Dec; 66(3):425–40.

28. Eby, G. A., et al. Reduction in duration of common colds by zinc gluconate lozenges in a double-blind study. *Antimicrob Agents Chemother* 1984 Jan; 25(1):20–4.
29. Al-Nakib, W., et al. Prophylaxis and treatment of rhinovirus colds with zinc gluconate lozenges. *J Antimicrob Chemother* 1987 Dec; 20(6):893–901.
30. Mossad, S. B., et al. Zinc gluconate lozenges for treating the common cold. A randomized, double-blind, placebo-controlled study. *Ann Intern Med* 1996 Jul 15; 125(2):81–88.
31. Gaby, A. R., Wright, J. V. Nutritional factors in degenerative eye disorders: cataract and macular degeneration. *J Adv Med* 1993 Spring; 6(1):27–40.
32. Knekt, P., Marniemi, J., Teppo, L., Heliovaara, M., Aromaa, A. Is low selenium status a risk factor for lung cancer? *Am J Epidemiol* 1998 Nov 15; 148(10):975–82.
33. Clark, L. C., Combs, G. F., Jr., Turnbull, B. W., et al. Effects of selenium supplementation for cancer prevention in patients with carcinoma of the skin. A randomized controlled trial. Nutritional Prevention of Cancer Study Group. *JAMA* 1996 Dec 25; 276(24):1957–63.
34. Clark, L. C., Dalkin, B., Krongrad, A., et al. Decreased incidence of prostate cancer with selenium supplementation: results of a double-blind cancer prevention trial. *Br J Urol* 1998 May; 81(5):730–34.
35. Combs, G. F., Jr., Gray, W. P. Chemopreventive agents: selenium. *Pharmacol Ther* 1998 Sep; 79(3):179–92.
36. Ip, C., Lisk, D. J. Efficacy of cancer prevention by high-selenium garlic is primarily dependent on the action of selenium. *Carcinogenesis* 1995 Nov; 16(11):2649–52.
37. Chan, S., Gerson, B., Subramaniam, S. The role of copper, molybdenum, selenium, and zinc in nutrition and health. *Clin Lab Med* 1998 Dec; 18(4):673–85.
38. Anderson, R. A., Polansky, M. M., Bryden, N. A., Roginski E.E., Mertz W., Glinsmann W. Chromium supplementation of human subjects: effects on glucose, insulin, and lipid variables. *Metabolism* 32(9):894–99 Sep 1983.

39. Anderson, R. A. Chromium and parenteral nutrition. Nutrition 1995 Jan–Feb; 11(1 Suppl):83–86.

40. Anderson, R. A. Recent advances in the clinical and biochemical effects of chromium deficiency. *Prog Clin Biol Res* 1993; 380:221–34.

41. Stearns, D. M., Belbruno, J. J., Wetterhahn, K. E. A prediction of chromium (III) accumulation in humans from chromium dietary supplements. *FASEB J* 1995 Dec; 9(15):1650–57.

42. Clancy, S. P., Clarkson, P. M., DeCheke, M. E., et al. Effects of chromium picolinate supplementation on body composition, strength, and urinary chromium loss in football players. *Int J Sport Nutr* 1994 Jun; 4(2):142–53.

43. Lee, N. A., Reasner, C. A. Beneficial effect of chromium supplementation on serum triglyceride levels in NIDDM. *Diabetes Care* 1994 Dec; 17(12):1449–52.

44. Morris, B. W., Blumsohn, A., Mac Neil, S., Gray, T. A. The trace element chromium—a role in glucose homeostasis. *Am J Clin Nutr* 1992 May; 55(5):989–91.

45. Mahdi, G. S. Chromium in barley potentiates insulin [letter; comment]. *Am J Clin Nutr* 1995 Mar; 61(3):614–15.

46. Anderson, R. A., Cheng, N., Bryden, N. A., et al. Beneficial effects of chromium for people with type II Diabetes. *Diabetes* 45:124A, 1996.

47. Salonen, J. T., Nyyssonen, K., Korpela, H., et al. High stored iron levels are associated with excess risk of myocardial infarction in eastern Finnish men. *Circulation* 1992 Sep; 86(3):803–11.

48. Ascherio, A., Willett, W. C., Rimm, E. B. et al. Dietary iron intake and risk of coronary disease among men. *Circulation* 1994 Mar; 89(3):969–74.

49. Meyers, D. G., Strickland, D., Maloley, P. A., et al. Possible association of a reduction in cardiovascular events with blood donation. *Heart* 1997 Aug; 78(2):188–93.

50. Volpe, S. L., Taper, L. J., Meacham, S. The relationship between boron and magnesium status and bone mineral density in the human: a review. *Magnes Res* 1993 Sep; 6(3):291–96.

51. Nielsen, F. H. Studies on the relationship between boron and magnesium which possibly affects the formation and maintenance of bones. *Magnes Trace Elem* 1990; 9(2):61–69.
52. Joshi, P. C. Copper (II) as an efficient scavenger of singlet molecular oxygen. *Indian J Biochem Biophys* 1998 Aug; 35(4):208–15.
53. Giovanetti, A., Rossi, L., Mancuso, M., et al. Analysis of lung damage induced by trichloroethylene inhalation in mice fed diets with low, normal, and high copper content. *Toxicol Pathol* 1998 Sep–Oct; 26(5):628–35.

Chapter 6. *Dietary Fats and Essential Fatty Acids*

1. Simopoulos, A. P. Omega-3 fatty acids in health and disease and in growth and development. *Am J Clin Nutr* 1991 Sep; 54(3):438–63.
2. Koletzko, B. Trans fatty acids may impair biosynthesis of long-chain polyunsaturates and growth in man. *Acta Paediatr* 1992 Apr; 81(4):302–6.
3. Kohlmeier, L. Biomarkers of fatty acid exposure and breast cancer risk. *Am J Clin Nutr* 1997 Dec; 66(6 Suppl):1548S–1556S.
4. Booyens, J., van der Merwe, C. F. Margarines and coronary artery disease. *Med Hypotheses* 1992 Apr; 37(4):241–44.
5. Pedersen, J. I., Johansson, L., Thelle, D. S. Trans-fatty acids and health. *Tidsskr Nor Laegeforen* 1998 Sep 20; 118(22):3474–80.
6. Rudin, D. O. The dominant diseases of modernized societies as omega-3 essential fatty acid deficiency syndrome: substrate beriberi. *Med Hypotheses* 1982 Jan; 8(1):17–47.
7. Rudin, D. O. The major psychoses and neuroses as omega-3 essential fatty acid deficiency syndrome: substrate pellagra. *Biol Psychiatry* 1981 Sep; 16(9):837–50.
8. Ponte, E., Cafagna, D., Balbi, M. Cardiovascular disease and omega-3 fatty acids. *Minerva Med* 1997 Sep; 88(9):343–53.
9. Morcos, N. C. Modulation of lipid profile by fish oil and garlic combination. *J Natl Med Assoc* 1997 Oct; 89(10):673–78.
10. Hu, F. B., Stampfer, M. J., Manson, J. E., et al. Dietary fat intake and the risk of coronary heart disease in women. *N Engl J Med* 1997; 337:1491–99.

11. Albert, C. M., Hennekens, C. H., O'Donnell, C. J., et al. Fish consumption and risk of sudden cardiac death. *JAMA* 1998 Jan; 279:23–28.
12. Mori, T. A., et al. The effects of fish and fish oils on platelet function in men at risk of coronary heart disease. *Arterioscler Thromb Vasc Biol* 1997; 17:279–86.
13. Kim, D. N., Eastman, A., Baker, J. E., et al. Fish oil, atherogenesis, and thrombogenesis. *Ann N Y Acad Sci* 1995 Jan 17; 748:474–80.
14. Belch, J. J., Ansell, D., Madhok, R., O'Dowd, A., Sturrock, R. D. Effects of altering dietary essential fatty acids on requirements for non-steroidal anti-inflammatory drugs in patients with rheumatoid arthritis: a double blind placebo controlled study. *Ann Rheum Dis* 1988 Feb; 47(2):96–104.
15. Heller, A., Koch, T., Schmeck, J., van Ackern, K. Lipid mediators in inflammatory disorders. *Drugs* 1998 Apr; 55(4):487–96.
16. Khalfoun, B., Thibault, G., Bardos, P., Lebranchu, Y. Docosahexaenoic and eicosapentaenoic acids inhibit in vitro human lymphocyte-endothelial cell adhesion. *Transplantation* 1996 Dec 15; 62(11):1649–57.
17. Otto, D. A., Kahn, D. R., Hamm, M. W., Forrest, D. E., Wooten, J. T. Improved survival of heterotopic cardiac allografts in rats with dietary n-3 polyunsaturated fatty acids. *Transplantation* 1990 Aug; 50(2):193–98.
18. Stenson, W. F., Cort, D., Rodgers, J., et al. Dietary supplementation with fish oil in ulcerative colitis. *Ann Intern Med* 1992 Apr 15; 116(8):609–14.
19. Galland, L. Increased requirements for essential fatty acids in atopic individuals: a review with clinical descriptions. *J Am Coll Nutr* 1986; 5(2):213–28.
20. Kojima, T., Terano, T., Tanabe, E., Okamoto, S., Tamura, Y., Yoshida, S. Long-term administration of highly purified eicosapentaenoic acid provides improvement of psoriasis. *Dermatologica* 1991; 182(4):225–30.
21. Arm, J. P., and Lee, T. H. The use of fish oil in bronchial asthma. *Allergy Proc* 1989 May–Jun; 10(3):185–87.
22. Hashimoto, N., Majima, T., Ichimura, K., Iwata, T., Suguro, H., Horie, T. Effects of eicosapentaenoic acid in patients with bronchial asthma. *Nihon Kyobu Shikkan Gakkai Zasshi* 1997 Jun; 35(6):634–40.

23. Kikuchi, S., Sakamoto, T., Ishikawa, C., Yazawa, K., Torii, S. Modulation of eosinophil chemotactic activities to leukotriene B_4 by n-3 polyunsaturated fatty acids. *Prostaglandins Leukot Essent Fatty Acids* 1998 Mar; 58(3):243–48.

24. Thompson, L. U., Rickard, S. E., Orcheson, L. J., Seidl, M. M. Flaxseed and its lignan and oil components reduce mammary tumor growth at a late stage of carcinogenesis. *Carcinogenesis* 1996 Jun; 17(6):1373–76.

25. Christophe, A., Robberecht, E., Franckx, H., De Baets, F., van de Pas, M. Effect of administration of gamma-linolenic acid on the fatty acid composition of serum phospholipids and cholesteryl esters in patients with cystic fibrosis. *Ann Nutr Metab* 1994; 38(1):40–47.

26. Engler, M. M. Comparative study of diets enriched with evening primrose, black currant, borage or fungal oils on blood pressure and pressor responses in spontaneously hypertensive rats. *Prostaglandins Leukot Essent Fatty Acids* 1993 Oct; 49(4):809–14.

27. Leventhal, L. J., Boyce, E. G., Zurier, R. B. Treatment of rheumatoid arthritis with gammalinolenic acid. *Ann Intern Med* 1993 Nov 1; 119(9):867–73.

28. Raederstorff, D., Moser, U. Borage or primrose oil added to standardized diets are equivalent sources for gamma-linolenic acid in rats. *Lipids* 1992 Dec; 27(12):1018–23.

29. Bahmer, F. A., Schafer, J. Treatment of atopic dermatitis with borage seed oil (Glandol)—a time series analytic study. *Kinderarztl Prax* 1992 Oct; 60(7):199–202.

30. Pullman-Mooar, S., Laposata, M., Lem, D., et al. Alteration of the cellular fatty acid profile and the production of eicosanoids in human monocytes by gamma-linolenic acid. *Arthritis Rheum* 1990 Oct; 33(10):1526–33.

31. Tate, G., Mandell, B. F., Laposata, M., et al. Suppression of acute and chronic inflammation by dietary gamma linolenic acid. *J Rheumatol* 1989 Jun; 16(6):729–34.

32. Horrobin, D. F., and Manku, M. S. Premenstrual syndrome and premenstrual breast pain (cyclical mastalgia): disorders of essential fatty

acid (EFA) metabolism. *Prostaglandins Leukot Essent Fatty Acids* 1989 Sep; 37(4):255–61.

33. Mills, D. E., Prkachin, K. M., Harvey, K. A., Ward, R. P. Dietary fatty acid supplementation alters stress reactivity and performance in man. *J Hum Hypertens* 1989 Apr; 3(2):111–16.
34. Miller, C. C., and Ziboh, V. A. Gammalinolenic acid-enriched diet alters cutaneous eicosanoids. *Biochem Biophys Res Commun* 1988 Aug 15; 154(3):967–74.
35. Horrobin, D. F. Essential fatty acid and prostaglandin metabolism in Sjögren's syndrome, systemic sclerosis and rheumatoid arthritis. *Scand J Rheumatol Suppl* 1986; 61:242–45.
36. Begin, M. E., Ells, G., Das, U. N., Horrobin, D. F. Differential killing of human carcinoma cells supplemented with n-3 and n-6 polyunsaturated fatty acids. *J Natl Cancer Inst* 1986 Nov; 77(5):1053–62.

Chapter 7. Amino Acids and Hormones

1. Hill, R. H., Jr., Caudill, S. P., et al. Contaminants in L-tryptophan associated with eosinophilia myalgia syndrome. *Arch Environ Contam Toxicol* 1993 Jul; 25(1):134–42.
2. Slutsker, L., Hoesly, F. C., et al. Eosinophilia-myalgia syndrome associated with exposure to tryptophan from a single manufacturer. *JAMA* 1990 Jul 11; 264(2):213–17.
3. Philen, R. M., Hill, R. H., Jr., et al. Tryptophan contaminants associated with eosinophilia-myalgia syndrome. The Eosinophilia-Myalgia Studies of Oregon, New York and New Mexico. *Am J Epidemiol* 1993 Aug 1; 138(3):154–59.
4. Takagi, H., Ochoa, M. S., et al. Enhanced collagen synthesis and transcription by peak E, a contaminant of L-tryptophan preparations associated with the eosinophilia myalgia syndrome epidemic. *J Clin Invest* 1995 Nov; 96(5):2120–25.
5. Lacey, J. M., Wilmore, D. W. Is glutamine a conditionally essential amino acid? *Nutr Rev* 1990 Aug; 48(8):297–309.
6. Harward, T. R., Coe, D., Souba, W. W., Klingman, N., Seeger, J. M. Glutamine preserves gut glutathione levels during intestinal ischemia/reperfusion. *J Surg Res* 1994 Apr; 56(4):351–55.

7. Souba, W. W., Klimberg, V. S., Plumley, D. A., et al. The role of glutamine in maintaining a healthy gut and supporting the metabolic response to injury and infection. *J Surg Res* 1990 Apr; 48(4):383–91.
8. Souba, W.W. Glutamine and cancer. *Ann Surg* 1993 Dec; 218(6):715–28.
9. Rouse, K., Nwokedi, E., Woodliff, J. E., et al. Glutamine enhances selectivity of chemotherapy through changes in glutathione metabolism. *Ann Surg* 1995; 221:420–26.
10. Li, J., Langkamp-Henken, B., Suzuki, K., Stahlgren, L. H. Glutamine prevents parenteral nutrition-induced increases in intestinal permeability. *JPEN J Parenter Enteral Nutr* 1994; 18:303–7.
11. Pola, P., et al. Statistical evaluation of long-term L-carnitine therapy in hyperlipoproteinaemias. *Drugs Exptl Clin Res* 1983; 9:925–34.
12. Orlando, G., Rusconi, C. Oral L-carnitine in the treatment of chronic cardiac ischaemia in elderly patients. *Clin Trials J* 1986; 23:338–44.
13. Singh, R. B., Niaz, M. A., et al. A randomised, double-blind, placebo-controlled trial of L-carnitine in suspected acute myocardial infarction. *Postgrad Med J* 1996 Jan; 72(843):45–50.
14. Kamikawa, T., Suzuki, Y., Kobayashi, A., et al. Effects of L-carnitine on exercise tolerance in patients with stable angina pectoris. *Jpn Heart J* 1984 Jul; 25(4):587–97.
15. Siliprandi, N., Di Lisa, F., Toninello, A. Biochemical derangements in ischemic myocardium: the role of carnitine. *G Ital Cardiol* 1984 Oct; 14(10):804–8.
16. Kobayashi, A., Watanabe, H., et al. Effects of L-carnitine and palmitoylcarnitine on membrane fluidity of human erythrocytes. *Biochim Biophys Acta* 1989 Nov; 986(1):83–88.
17. Ghidini, O., Azzurro, M., Vita, G., Sartori, G. Evaluation of the therapeutic efficacy of L-carnitine in congestive heart failure. *Int J Clin Pharmacol Ther Toxicol* 1988 Apr; 26(4):217–20.
18. Cherchi, A., Lai, C., Angelino, F., et al. Effects of L-carnitine on exercise tolerance in chronic stable angina: a multicenter, double-blind, randomized, placebo controlled crossover study. *Int J Clin Pharmacol Ther Toxicol* 1985 Oct; 23(10):569–72.

19. Scholte, H. R., Luyt-Houwen, I. E., Vaandrager-Verduin, M. H. The role of the carnitine system in myocardial fatty acid oxidation:carnitine deficiency, failing mitochondria and cardiomyopathy. *Basic Res Cardiol* 1987; 82 Suppl 1:63–73.
20. Greig, C., Finch, K. M., Jones, D. A., Cooper, M., Sargeant, A. J., Forte, C. A. The effect of oral supplementation with L-carnitine on maximum and submaximum exercise capacity. *Eur J Appl Physiol* 1987; 56(4):457–60.
21. Dragan, I. G., and Vasiliu, A., et al. Studies concerning chronic and acute effects of L-carnitina in elite athletes. *Physiologie* 1989 Apr–Jun; 26(2):111–29.
22. Marconi, C., Sassi, G., Carpinelli, A., Cerretelli, P. Effects of L-carnitine loading on the aerobic and anaerobic performance of endurance athletes. *Eur J Appl Physiol* 1985; 54(2):131–35.
23. Fischer, E., Heller, B., Nachon, M., Spatz, H. Therapy of depression by phenylalanine. Preliminary note. *Arzneimittelforschung* 1975 Jan; 25(1):132.
24. Beckmann, H., Athen, D., Olteanu, M., Zimmer, R. DL-phenylalanine versus imipramine: a double-blind controlled study. *Arch Psychiatr Nervenkr* 1979 Jul 4; 227(1):49–58.
25. Beckmann, H., and Ludolph, E. DL-phenylalanine as an antidepressant. Open study. *Arzneimittelforschung* 1978; 28(8):1283–84.
26. Birkmayer, W., Riederer, P., Linauer, W., Knoll, J. L-deprenyl plus L-phenylalanine in the treatment of depression. *J Neural Transm* 1984; 59(1):81–87.
27. Hishikawa, K., Nakaki, T., Tsuda, M., et al. Effect of systemic L-arginine administration on hemodynamics and nitric oxide release in man. *Jpn Heart J* 1992 Jan; 33(1):41–48.
28. Loscalzo, J. Nitric oxide in vascular disease. *N Engl J Med* 1995 July 27; 333(4):251–53.
29. Bode-Boger, S. M., Boger, R. H., Alfke, H., et al. L-arginine induces nitric oxide-dependent vasodilation in patients with critical limb ischemia. A randomized, controlled study. *Circulation* 1996 Jan 1; 93(1):85–90.

30. Rector, T. S., et al. Randomized, double-blind, placebo-controlled study of supplemental oral L-arginine in patients with heart failure. *Circulation* 1996 Jun 15; 93(12):2135–41.

31. Adams, M. R., McCredie, R., Jessup, W., et al. Oral L-arginine improves endothelium-dependent dilatation and reduces monocyte adhesion to endothelial cells in young men with coronary artery disease. *Atherosclerosis* 1997 Mar 21; 129(2):261–69.

32. Bellamy, M. F., Goodfellow, J., Tweddel, A. C., et al. Syndrome X and endothelial dysfunction. *Cardiovasc Res* 1998 Nov; 40(2):410–17.

33. Barbul, A., Lazarou, S. A., Efron, D. T., Wasserkrug, H. L., Efron, G. Arginine enhances wound healing and lymphocyte immune responses in humans. *Surgery* 1990 Aug; 108(2):331–36.

34. Chuntrasakul, C., Siltharm, S., Sarasombath, S., et al. Metabolic and immune effects of dietary arginine, glutamine and omega-3 fatty acids supplementation in immunocompromised patients. *J Med Assoc Thai* 1998 May; 81(5):334–43.

35. Baligan, M., Giardina, A., Giovannini, G., et al. L-arginine and immunity. Study of pediatric subjects. *Minerva Pediatr* 1997 Nov; 49(11):537–42.

36. Moody, J. A., Vernet, D., Laidlaw, S., et al. Effects of long-term oral administration of L-arginine on the rat erectile response. *J Urol* 1997 Sep; 158(3 Pt 1):942–47.

37. Griffith, R. S., et al. Success of L-lysine therapy in frequently recurrent herpes simplex infection. *Dermatologica,* 1987; 175:183–90.

38. McCune, M. A., et al. Treatment of recurrent herpes simplex infections with L-lysine monohydrochloride. *Cutis* 1984; 34(4): 366–73.

39. Milman, N., et al. Lysine prophylaxis in recurrent herpes simplex labialis: A double-blind, crossover study. *Acta Dermatovener,* 1980; 60:85–87.

40. Pauling, L. Case Report: Lysine/Ascorbate-Related Amelioration of Angina Pectoris, *J Orthomol Med Soc,* 1991; 6(3&4):144–46.

41. Harpel, P. C., Borth, W. Identification of mechanisms that may modulate the role of lipoprotein (a) in thrombosis and atherogenesis, *Ann Epidemiol,* 1992, Jul; 2(4):413–17.

42. Chesney, R. W. Taurine: its biological role and clinical implications. *Adv Pediatr* 1985; 32:1–42.
43. Pisarenko, O. I. Mechanisms of myocardial protection by amino acids: facts and hypotheses. *Clin Exp Pharmacol Physiol* 1996 Aug; 23(8):627–33.
44. Azuma, J., et al. Beneficial effect of taurine on congestive heart failure induced by chronic aortic regurgitation in rabbits. *Res Commun Chem Pathol Pharmacol* 1984 Aug; 45(2):261–70.
45. Azuma, J., et al. Taurine for treatment of congestive heart failure. *Int J Cardiol* 1982; 2(2):303–4.
46. Azuma, J., et al. Therapeutic effect of taurine in congestive heart failure: a double-blind crossover trial. *Clin Cardiol* 1985 May; 8(5):276–82.
47. Fujita, T., Sato, Y. Hypotensive effect of taurine. Possible involvement of the sympathetic nervous system and endogenous opiates. *J Clin Invest* 1988 Sep; 82(3):993–97.
48. Gaby, A. R., Wright, J. V. Nutritional factors in degenerative eye disorders: cataract and macular degeneration. *J Adv Med* 1993 Spring; 6(1):27–40.
49. Van Gelder, N. M., Koyama. I., Jasper. H. H. Taurine treatment of spontaneous chronic epilepsy in a cat. *Epilepsia* 1977 Mar; 18(1):45–54.
50. Durelli, L., Mutani, R., Fassio, F., Satta, A., Bartoli, E. Taurine and hyperexcitable human muscle: effects of taurine on potassium-induced hyperexcitability of dystrophic myotonic and normal muscles. *Ann Neurol* 1982 Mar; 11(3):258–65.
51. Smith, K. A., et al. (As reported in Reuter's Medical News), *Arch Gen Psychiatry* 1999; 56:171–76.
52. Angst, J., Woggon, B., Schoepf, J. The treatment of depression with L-5-hydroxytryptophan versus imipramine. Results of two open and one double-blind study. *Arch Psychiatr Nervenkr* 1977 Oct 11; 224(2):175–86.
53. Nardini, M., De Stefano, R., Iannuccelli, M., Borghesi, R., Battistini, N. Treatment of depression with L-5-hydroxytryptophan combined with chlorimipramine, a double-blind study. *Int J Clin Pharmacol Res* 1983; 3(4):239–50.

54. Caruso, I., Sarzi Puttini, P., Cazzola, M., Azzolini, V. Double-blind study of 5-hydroxytryptophan versus placebo in the treatment of primary fibromyalgia syndrome. *J Int Med Res* 1990 May–Jun; 18(3):201–9.
55. Longo, G., Rudoi, I., Iannuccelli, M., Strinati, R., Panizon, F. Treatment of essential headache in developmental age with L-5-HTP (cross over double-blind study versus placebo). *Pediatr Med Chir* 1984 Mar–Apr; 6(2):241–45.
56. Titus, F., Davalos, A., Alom, J., Codina, A. 5-Hydroxytryptophan versus methysergide in the prophylaxis of migraine. Randomized clinical trial. *Eur Neurol* 1986; 25(5):327–29.

Chapter 8. *Flavonoids, Herbs, and Botanicals*

1. Saija, A., Scalese, M., Lanza, M., et al. Flavonoids as antioxidant agents: importance of their interaction with biomembranes. *Free Radic Biol Med* 1995 Oct; 19(4):481–86.
2. Lietti, A., Cristoni, A., Picci, M. Studies on Vaccinium myrtillus anthocyanosides. I. Vasoprotective and antiinflammatory activity. *Arzneimittelforschung* 1976; 26(5):829–32.
3. Detre, Z., Jellinek, H., Miskulin, M., Robert, A. M. Studies on vascular permeability in hypertension: action of anthocyanosides. *Clin Physiol Biochem* 1986; 4(2):143–49.
4. Bomser, J., Madhavi, D. L., Singletary, K., Smith, M. A. In vitro anticancer activity of fruit extracts from Vaccinium species. *Planta Med* 1996 Jun; 62(3):212–16.
5. Laplaud, P. M., Lelubre, A., Chapman, M. J. Antioxidant action of Vaccinium myrtillus extract on human low density lipoproteins in vitro: initial observations. *Fundam Clin Pharmacol* 1997; 11(1):35–40.
6. Scharrer, A., Ober, M. Anthocyanosides in the treatment of retinopathies. *Klin Monatsbl Augenheilkd* 1981 May; 178(5):386–89.
7. Boniface, R., Robert, A. M. Effect of anthocyanins on human connective tissue metabolism in the human. *Klin Monatsbl Augenheilkd* 1996 Dec; 209(6):368–72.
8. Lieberman, S. A review of the effectiveness of Cimicifuga racemosa (black cohosh) for the symptoms of menopause. *J Womens Health* 1998 Jun; 7(5):525–29.

9. Liske, E. Therapeutic efficacy and safety of Cimicifuga racemosa for gynecologic disorders. *Adv Ther* 1998 Jan–Feb; 15(1):45–53.
10. Lehmann-Willenbrock, E., Riedel, H. H. [Clinical and endocrinologic studies of the treatment of ovarian insufficiency manifestations following hysterectomy with intact adnexa] *Zentralbl Gynakol* 1988; 110(10):611–18.
11. Fleet, J. C. New support for a folk remedy: cranberry juice reduces bacteriuria and pyuria in elderly women. *Nutr Rev* 1994 May; 52(5):168–70.
12. Avorn, J., Monane, M., Gurwitz, J. H., et al. Reduction of bacteriuria and pyuria after ingestion of cranberry juice. *JAMA* 1994 Mar 9; 271(10):751–54.
13. Zafriri, D., Ofek, I., Adar, R., Pocino, M., Sharon, N. Inhibitory activity of cranberry juice on adherence of type 1 and type P fimbriated Escherichia coli to eucaryotic cells. *Antimicrob Agents Chemother* 1989 Jan; 33(1):92–98.
14. Sobota, A. E. Inhibition of bacterial adherence by cranberry juice: potential use for the treatment of urinary tract infections. *J Urol* 1984 May; 131(5):1013–16.
15. Wilson, T., Porcari, J. P., Harbin, D. Cranberry extract inhibits low density lipoprotein oxidation. *Life Sci* 1998; 62(24):PL381–86.
16. See, D. M., Broumand, N., Sahl, L., Tilles, J. G. In vitro effects of echinacea and ginseng on natural killer and antibody-dependent cell cytotoxicity in healthy subjects and chronic fatigue syndrome or acquired immunodeficiency syndrome patients. *Immunopharmacology* 1997 Jan; 35(3):229–35.
17. Wildfeuer, A., and Mayerhofer, D. The effects of plant preparations on cellular functions in body defense. *Arzneimittelforschung* 1994 Mar; 44(3):361–66.
18. Bauer, V. R., Jurcic, K., Puhlmann, J., Wagner, H. Immunologic in vivo and in vitro studies on Echinacea extracts. *Arzneimittelforschung* 1988 Feb; 38(2):276–81.
19. Burger, R. A., Torres, A. R., Warren, R. P., Caldwell, V. D., Hughes, B. G. Echinacea-induced cytokine production by human macrophages. *Int J Immunopharmacol* 1997 Jul; 19(7):371–79.

20. Johnson, E. S., Kadam, N. P., Hylands, D. M., Hylands, P. J. Efficacy of feverfew as prophylactic treatment of migraine. *Br Med J* (Clin Res Ed) 1985 Aug 31; 291(6495):569–73.

21. Murphy, J. J., Heptinstall, S., Mitchell, J. R. Randomised double-blind placebo-controlled trial of feverfew in migraine prevention. *Lancet* 1988 Jul 23; 2(8604):189–92.

22. Sumner, H., Salan, U., Knight, D. W., Hoult, J. R. Inhibition of 5-lipoxygenase and cyclo-oxygenase in leukocytes by feverfew. Involvement of sesquiterpene lactones and other components. *Biochem Pharmacol* 1992 Jun 9; 43(11):2313–20.

23. Groenewegen, W. A., Heptinstall, S. A comparison of the effects of an extract of feverfew and parthenolide, a component of feverfew, on human platelet activity in-vitro. *J Pharm Pharmacol* 1990 Aug; 42(8):553–57.

24. Hayes, N. A., Foreman, J. C. The activity of compounds extracted from feverfew on histamine release from rat mast cells. *J Pharm Pharmacol* 1987 Jun; 39(6):466–70.

25. Loesche, W., Mazurov, A. V., et al. Feverfew—an antithrombotic drug? *Folia Haematol Int Mag Klin Morphol Blutforsch* 1988; 115(1–2):181–84.

26. Losche, W., Mazurov, A. V., Heptinstall, S., et al. An extract of feverfew inhibits interactions of human platelets with collagen substrates. *Thromb Res* 1987 Dec 1; 48(5):511–18.

27. Isensee, H., Rietz, B., Jacob, R. Cardioprotective actions of garlic (Allium sativum). *Arzneimittelforschung* 1993 Feb; 43(2):94–98.

28. Foushee, D. B., Ruffin, J., Banerjee, U. Garlic as a natural agent for the treatment of hypertension: a preliminary report. *Cytobios* 1982; 34(135–36):145–52.

29. Silagy, C. A., and Neil, H. A. A meta-analysis of the effect of garlic on blood pressure. *J Hypertens* 1994 Apr; 12(4):463–68.

30. Steiner, M., Khan, A. H., Holbert, D., Lin, R. I. A double-blind crossover study in moderately hypercholesterolemic men that compared the effect of aged garlic extract and placebo administration on blood lipids. *Am J Clin Nutr* 1996 Dec; 64(6):866–70.

31. Adler, A. J., and Holub, B. J. Effect of garlic and fish-oil supplementation on serum lipid and lipoprotein concentrations in hypercholesterolemic men. *Am J Clin Nutr* 1997 Feb; 65(2):445–50.
32. Bordia, A., Verma, S. K., Srivastava, K. C. Effect of garlic (Allium sativum) on blood lipids, blood sugar, fibrinogen and fibrinolytic activity in patients with coronary artery disease. *Prostaglandins Leukot Essent Fatty Acids* 1998 Apr; 58(4):257–63.
33. Milner, J. A. Garlic: its anticarcinogenic and antitumorigenic properties. *Nutr Rev* 1996 Nov; 54(11 Pt 2):S82–86.
34. Torok, B., Belagyi, J., Rietz, B., Jacob, R. Effectiveness of garlic on the radical activity in radical generating systems. *Arzneimittelforschung* 1994 May; 44(5):608–11.
35. Das, I., Khan, N. S., Sooranna, S. R. Potent activation of nitric oxide synthase by garlic: a basis for its therapeutic applications. *Curr Med Res Opin* 1995; 13(5):257–63.
36. Raloff, J. Aged garlic could slow prostate cancer. *Science News* 1997 April; 151:239.
37. Pai, S. T., and Platt, M. W. Antifungal effects of Allium sativum (garlic) extract against the Aspergillus species involved in otomycosis. *Lett Appl Microbiol* 1995 Jan; 20(1):14–18.
38. Yoshikawa, M., Yamaguchi, S., Kunimi, K., et al. Stomachic principles in ginger. III. An anti-ulcer principle, 6-gingesulfonic acid, and three monoacyldigalactosylglycerols, gingerglycolipids A, B, and C, from Zingiberis Rhizoma originating in Taiwan. *Chem Pharm Bull* (Tokyo) 1994 Jun; 42(6):1226–30.
39. Phillips, S., Ruggier, R., Hutchinson, S. E. Zingiber officinale (ginger)—an antiemetic for day case surgery. *Anaesthesia* 1993 Aug; 48(8):715–17.
40. Fischer-Rasmussen, W., Kjaer, S. K., Dahl, C., Asping, U. Ginger treatment of hyperemesis gravidarum. *Eur J Obstet Gynecol Reprod Biol* 1991 Jan 4; 38(1):19–24.
41. Bone, M.E., Wilkinson, D. J., Young, J. R., McNeil, J., Charlton S. Ginger root—a new antiemetic. The effect of ginger root on postoperative nausea and vomiting after major gynaecological surgery. *Anaesthesia* 1990 Aug; 45(8):669–71.

42. Sharma, J. N., Srivastava, K. C., Gan, E. K. Suppressive effects of eugenol and ginger oil on arthritic rats. *Pharmacology* 1994 Nov; 49(5):314–18.

43. Srivastava, K. C., Mustafa, T. Ginger (Zingiber officinale) in rheumatism and musculoskeletal disorders. *Med Hypotheses* 1992 Dec; 39(4):342–48.

44. Verma, S. K., Singh, J., Khamesra, R., Bordia, A. Effect of ginger on platelet aggregation in man. *Indian J Med Res* 1993 Oct; 98:240–42.

45. Le Bars, P. L., Katz, M. M., Berman, N., et al. A placebo-controlled, double-blind, randomized trial of an extract of ginkgo biloba for dementia. *JAMA* 1997 Oct; 278:1327–32.

46. Kleijnen, J., Knipschild, P. Ginkgo biloba, intermittent claudication and cerebral insufficiency. *Lancet* 1992 Nov; 340:1136–39.

47. Akiba, S., Kawauchi, T., Oka, T., Hashizume, T., Sato, T. Inhibitory effect of the leaf extract of Ginkgo biloba L. on oxidative stress-induced platelet aggregation. *Biochem Mol Biol Int* 1998 Dec; 46(6):1243–48.

48. Lee, S. L., Wang, W. W., Lanzillo, J., Gillis, C. N., Fanburg, B. L. Superoxide scavenging effect of Ginkgo biloba extract on serotonin-induced mitogenesis. *Biochem Pharmacol* 1998 Aug 15; 56(4):527–33.

49. Doly, M., Droy-Lefaix, M. T., Braquet, P. Oxidative stress in diabetic retina. *EXS* 1992; 62:299–307.

50. Cohen, A. J., and Bartlik, B. Ginkgo biloba for antidepressant-induced sexual dysfunction. *J Sex Marital Ther* 1998 Apr–Jun; 24(2):139–43.

51. Chen, X. Cardiovascular protection by ginsenosides and their nitric oxide releasing action. *Clin Exp Pharmacol Physiol* 1996 Aug; 23(8):728–32.

52. Han, K. H., Choe, S. C., Kim, H. S., et al. Effect of red ginseng on blood pressure in patients with essential hypertension and white coat hypertension. *Am J Chin Med* 1998; 26(2):199–209.

53. Ben-Hur, E., Fulder, S. Effect of Panax ginseng saponins and Eleutherococcus senticosus on survival of cultured mammalian cells after ionizing radiation. *Am J Chin Med* 1981 Spring; 9(1):48–56.

54. Bol'shakova, I. V., Lozovskaia, E. L., Sapezhinskii, I. I. Antioxidant properties of a series of extracts from medicinal plants. *Biofizika* 1997 Mar–Apr; 42(2):480–83.

55. Taik-Koo, Y., Soo-Yong, C. Non-organ specific cancer prevention of ginseng: a prospective study in Korea. *Int J Epidemiol* 1998 Jun; 27(3):359–64.
56. Singh, R. B., Niaz, M. A., Ghosh, S. Hypolipidemic and antioxidant effects of Commiphora mukul as an adjunct to dietary therapy in patients with hypercholesterolemia. *Cardiovasc Drugs Ther* 1994 Aug; 8(4):659–64.
57. Nityanand, S., Srivastava, J. S., Asthana, O. P. Clinical trials with gugulipid. A new hypolipidaemic agent. *J Assoc Physicians India* 1989 May; 37(5):323–28.
58. Thappa, D. M., and Dogra, J. Nodulocystic acne: oral gugulipid versus tetracycline. *J Dermatol* 1994 Oct; 21(10):729–31.
59. Leuchtgens, H. Crataegus special extract WS 1442 in NYHA II heart failure. A placebo controlled randomized double-blind study. *Fortschr Med* 1993 Jul; 111:352–54.
60. Blesken, R. Crataegus in cardiology. *Fortschr Med* 1992 May; 110:290–92.
61. Weihmayr, T., Ernst, E. Therapeutic effectiveness of Crataegus. *Fortschr Med* 1996 Jan; 114(1–2):27–29.
62. Volz, H. P., and Kieser, M. Kava-kava extract WS 1490 versus placebo in anxiety disorders—a randomized placebo-controlled 25-week outpatient trial. *Pharmacopsychiatry* 1997 Jan; 30(1):1–5.
63. Kinzler, E., Kromer, J., Lehmann, E. Effect of a special kava extract in patients with anxiety, tension, and excitation states of non-psychotic genesis. Double blind study with placebos over 4 weeks. *Arzneimittelforschung* 1991 Jun; 41(6):584–88.
64. Glick, L. Deglycyrrhizinated liquorice for peptic ulcer. *Lancet* 1982 Oct 9; 2(8302):817.
65. Bennett, A., Clark-Wibberley, T., Stamford, I. F., Wright, J. E. Aspirin-induced gastric mucosal damage in rats: cimetidine and deglycyrrhizinated liquorice together give greater protection than low doses of either drug alone. *J Pharm Pharmacol* 1980 Feb; 32(2):151.
66. Rees, W. D., Rhodes, J., Wright, J. E., Stamford, L. F., Bennett, A. Effect of deglycyrrhizinated liquorice on gastric mucosal damage by aspirin. *Scand J Gastroenterol* 1979; 14(5):605–7.

67. Lagrue, G., Olivier-Martin, F., Grillot, A. A study of the effects of procyanidol oligomers on capillary resistance in hypertension and in certain nephropathies. *Sem Hop* 1981 Sep 18–25; 57(33–36):1399–401.
68. Cheshier, J. E. Ardestani-Kaboudanian, S., Liang, B., et al., Immunomodulation by pycnogenol in retrovirus-infected or ethanol-fed mice. *Life Sci* 1996; 58(5): PL87–96.
69. Corbe, C., Boissin, J. P., Siou, A. Light vision and chorioretinal circulation. Study of the effect of procyanidolic oligomers (Endotelon). *J Fr Ophtalmol* 1988; 11(5):453–60.
70. Robert, L., Godeau, G., Gavignet-Jeannin, C., Groult, N., Six, C., Robert, A. M. The effect of procyanidolic oligomers on vascular permeability. A study using quantitative morphology. *Pathol Biol* (Paris) 1990 Jun; 38(6):608–16.
71. Pace-Asciak, C. R., Hahn, S., Diamandis, E. P., Soleas, G., Goldberg, D. M. The red wine phenolics trans-resveratrol and quercetin block human platelet aggregation and eicosanoid synthesis: implications for protection against coronary heart disease. *Clin Chim Acta* 1995 Mar 31; 235(2):207–19.
72. Ramanathan, R., Das, N. P., Tan, C. H. Effects of gamma-linolenic acid, flavonoids, and vitamins on cytotoxicity and lipid peroxidation. *Free Radic Biol Med* 1994 Jan; 16(1):43–48.
73. Formica, J. V., Regelson, W. Review of the biology of Quercetin and related bioflavonoids. *Food Chem Toxicol* 1995 Dec; 33(12):1061–80.
74. Champault, G., Patel, J. C., Bonnard, A. M. A double-blind trial of an extract of the plant Serenoa repens in benign prostatic hyperplasia. *Br J Clin Pharmacol* 1984 Sep; 18(3):461–62.
75. Champault, G., Bonnard, A. M., Cauquil, J., Patel, J. C. Actualite Therapeutique: The medical treatment of prostatic adenoma. *Ann Urol* 1984 Dec; 6:407–10.
76. Adriazola Semino, M., Lozano Ortega, J. L., et al. Symptomatic treatment of benign hypertrophy of the prostate. Comparative study of prazosin and serenoa repens. *Arch Esp Urol* 1992 Apr; 45(3):211–13.
77. Breu, W., Hagenlocher, M., Redl, K., Tittel, G., Stadler, F., Wagner, H. Anti-inflammatory activity of sabal fruit extracts prepared with supercritical carbon dioxide. In vitro antagonists of cyclooxygenase

and 5-lipoxygenase metabolism. *Arzneimittelforschung* 1992 Apr; 42(4):547–51.

78. Di Silverio, F., D'Eramo, G., et al. Evidence that Serenoa repens extract displays an antiestrogenic activity in prostatic tissue of benign prostatic hypertrophy patients. *Eur Urol* 1992; 21(4):309–14.
79. Grasso, M., Montesano, A., et al. Comparative effects of alfuzosin versus Serenoa repens in the treatment of symptomatic benign prostatic hyperplasia. *Arch Esp Urol* 1995 Jan–Feb; 48(1):97–103.
80. Di Silverio, F., D'Eramo, G., et al. Pharmacological combinations in the treatment of benign prostatic hypertrophy. *J Urol* (Paris) 1993; 99(6):316–20.
81. Strauch, G., Perles, P., Vergult, G., Gabriel, M., Gibelin, B., Cummings, S., Malbecq, W., Malice, M. P. Comparison of finasteride (Proscar) and Serenoa repens (Permixon) in the inhibition of 5-alpha reductase in healthy male volunteers. *Eur Urol* 1994; 26(3):247–52.
82. Plosker, G. L., Brogden, R. N. Serenoa repens (Permixon). A review of its pharmacology and therapeutic efficacy in benign prostatic hyperplasia. *Drugs Aging* 1996 Nov; 9(5):379–95.
83. Schneider, H. J., Honold, E., Masuhr, T. Treatment of benign prostatic hyperplasia. Results of a treatment study with the phytogenic combination of Sabal extract WS 1473 and Urtica extract WS 1031 in urologic specialty practices. *Fortschr Med* 1995 Jan 30; 113(3):37–40.
84. Krzeski, T., Kazon, M., Borkowski, A., Witeska, A., Kuczera, J. Combined extracts of Urtica dioica and Pygeum africanum in the treatment of benign prostatic hyperplasia: double-blind comparison of two doses. *Clin Ther* 1993 Nov–Dec; 15(6):1011–20.
85. Carani, C., Salvioli, V., Scuteri, A., Borelli, A., Baldini, A., Granata, A. R., Marrama, P. Urological and sexual evaluation of treatment of benign prostatic disease using Pygeum africanum at high doses. *Arch Ital Urol Nefrol Androl* 1991 Sep; 63(3):341–45.
86. Barlet, A., Albrecht, J., Aubert, A., et al. Efficacy of Pygeum africanum extract in the medical therapy of urination disorders due to benign prostatic hyperplasia: evaluation of objective and subjective parameters. A placebo-controlled double-blind multicenter study. *Wien Klin Wochenschr* 1990 Nov 23; 102(22):667–73.

87. Lang, I., Deak, G., Nekam, K., et al. Hepatoprotective and immunomodulatory effects of antioxidant therapy. *Acta Med Hung* 1988; 45(3–4):287–95.
88. Luper, S. A review of plants used in the treatment of liver disease: part 1. *Altern Med Rev* 1998 Dec; 3(6):410–21.
89. Feher, J., Lengyel, G., Blazovics, A. Oxidative stress in the liver and biliary tract diseases. *Scand J Gastroenterol Suppl* 1998; 228:38–46.
90. Skottova, N., Krecman, V. Silymarin as a potential hypocholesterolaemic drug. *Physiol Res* 1998; 47(1):1–7.
91. Sommer, H., Harrer, G. Placebo-controlled double-blind study examining the effectiveness of an hypericum preparation in 105 mildly depressed patients. *J Geriatr Psychiatry Neurol* 1994 Oct; 7 Suppl 1:S9–11.
92. Muller, W. E., Rossol, R. Effects of hypericum extract on the expression of serotonin receptors. *J Geriatr Psychiatry Neurol* 1994 Oct; 7 Suppl 1:S63–64.
93. Harrer, G., Schulz, V. Clinical investigation of the antidepressant effectiveness of hypericum. *J Geriatr Psychiatry Neurol* 1994 Oct; 7 Suppl 1:S6–8.
94. Mittman, P. Randomized, double-blind study of freeze-dried Urtica dioica in the treatment of allergic rhinitis. *Planta Med* 1990 Feb; 56(1):44–47.

Chapter 9. *Accessory Supplements*

1. Walaszek, Z., Szemraj, J., Narog, M., et al. Metabolism, uptake, and excretion of a D-glucaric acid salt and its potential use in cancer prevention. *Cancer Detect Prev* 1997; 21(2):178–90.
2. Webb, T. E., Pham-Nguyen, M. H., Darby, M., Hamme, A. T. 2nd, Pharmacokinetics relevant to the anti-carcinogenic and anti-tumor activities of glucarate and the synergistic combination of glucarate:retinoid in the rat. *Biochem Pharmacol* 1994 Apr 29; 47(9):1655–60.
3. Curley, R. W., Jr., Humphries, K. A., Koolemans-Beynan, A., et al. Activity of D-glucarate analogues: synergistic antiproliferative effects with retinoid in cultured human mammary tumor cells appear to

specifically require the D-glucarate structure. *Life Sci* 1994; 54(18):1299–303.

4. Webb, T. E., Abou-Issa, H., Stromberg, P. C., et al. Mechanism of growth inhibition of mammary carcinomas by glucarate and the glucarate:retinoid combination. *Anticancer Res* 1993 Nov–Dec; 13(6A):2095–99.
5. Abou-Issa, H., Dwivedi, C., Curley, R. W., Jr., et al. Basis for the anti-tumor and chemopreventive activities of glucarate and the glucarate:retinoid combination. *Anticancer Res* 1993 Mar–Apr; 13(2):395–99.
6. Heerdt, A. S., Young, C. W., Borgen, P. I. Calcium glucarate as a chemopreventive agent in breast cancer. *Isr J Med Sci* 1995 Feb–Mar; 31(2–3):101–5
7. Matsumura, T., Saji, S., Nakamura, R., Folkers, K. Evidence for enhanced treatment of periodontal disease by therapy with coenzyme Q. *Int J Vitam Nutr Res* 1973 Apr; 43(4):537–48.
8. Wilkinson, E. G., Arnold, R. M., Folkers, K. Bioenergetics in clinical medicine. VI. adjunctive treatment of periodontal disease with coenzyme Q_{10}. *Res Commun Chem Pathol Pharmacol* 1976 Aug; 14(4):715–19.
9. Hanioka, T., Tanaka, M., Ojima, M., Shizukuishi, S., Folkers, K. Effect of topical application of coenzyme Q_{10} on adult periodontitis. *Mol Aspects Med* 1994; 15 Suppl:s241–8.
10. Chello, M., Mastroroberto, P., Romano, R., et al. Protection by coenzyme Q_{10} from myocardial reperfusion injury during coronary artery bypass grafting. *Ann Thorac Surg* 1994 Nov; 58(5):1427–32.
11. Hano, O., Thompson-Gorman, S. L., Zweier, J. L., Lakatta, E. G. Coenzyme Q_{10} enhances cardiac functional and metabolic recovery and reduces Ca2+ overload during postischemic reperfusion. *Am J Physiol* 1994 Jun; 266(6 Pt 2):H2174–81.
12. Sanbe, A., Tanonaka, K., Niwano, Y., Takeo, S., Improvement of cardiac function and myocardial energy metabolism of rats with chronic heart failure by long-term coenzyme Q_{10} treatment. *J Pharmacol Exp Ther* 1994 Apr; 269(1):51–56.

13. Lelli, J. L., Drongowski R, A., Gastman, B., Remick, D. G., Coran, A. G. Effects of coenzyme Q_{10} on the mediator cascade of sepsis. *Circ Shock* 1993 Mar; 39(3):178–87.

14. Folkers, K., Morita, M., McRee, J., Jr. The activities of coenzyme Q_{10} and vitamin B_6 for immune responses. *Biochem Biophys Res Commun* 1993 May 28; 193(1):88–92.

15. Baggio, E., Gandini, R., Plancher, A. C., Passeri, M., Carmosino, G. Italian multicenter study on the safety and efficacy of coenzyme Q_{10} as adjunctive therapy in heart failure (interim analysis). The CoQ_{10} Drug Surveillance Investigators. *Clin Investig* 1993; 71(8 Suppl):S145–49.

16. Langsjoen, P., Langsjoen, P., Willis, R., Folkers, K. Treatment of essential hypertension with coenzyme Q_{10}. *Mol Aspects Med* 1994; 15 Suppl:S265–72.

17. Digiesi, V., Cantini, F., Oradei, A., et al. Coenzyme Q_{10} in essential hypertension. *Mol Aspects Med* 1994; 15 Suppl:S257–63.

18. Langsjoen, H., Langsjoen, P., Langsjoen, P., Willis, R., Folkers, K. Usefulness of coenzyme Q_{10} in clinical cardiology: a long-term study. *Mol Aspects Med* 1994; 15 Suppl:S165–75.

19. Langsjoen, P. H., and Langsjoen, A. M. Review of coenzyme Q_{10} in cardiovascular disease with emphasis on heart failure and ischemia reperfusion. *Asia Pacific Heart J.* 1998; 7(3):160–68.

20. Jesse, R. L., Loesser, K., Eich, D. M., et al. Dehydroepiandrosterone inhibits human platelet aggregation in vitro and in vivo. *Ann N Y Acad Sci* 1995 Dec 29; 774:281–90.

21. Slowinska-Srzednicka, J., et al. Hyperinsulinaemia and decreased plasma levels of dehydroepiandrosterone sulfate in premenopausal women with coronary heart disease. *J Intern Med* 1995 May; 237(5):465–72.

22. Simile, M., et al. Inhibition by dehydroepiandrosterone of growth and progression of persistent liver nodules in experimental rat liver carcinogenesis. *Int J Cancer* 1995 Jul 17; 62(2):210–15.

23. Kim, H. R., et al. Administration of dehydroepiandrosterone reverses the immune suppression induced by high dose antigen in mice. *Immunol Invest* 1995 May; 24(4):583–93.

24. Herrington, D. M. Dehydroepiandrosterone and coronary atherosclerosis. *Ann N Y Acad Sci* 1995 Dec 29; 774:271–80.
25. Schwartz, A. G., Pashko, L. L. Cancer prevention with dehydroepiandrosterone and non-androgenic structural analogs. *J Cell Biochem Suppl* 1995; 22:210–17.
26. Regelson, W., and Kalimi, M. Dehydroepiandrosterone (DHEA)—the multifunctional steroid. II. Effects on the CNS, cell proliferation, metabolic and vascular, clinical and other effects. Mechanism of action? *Ann N Y Acad Sci* 1994 May 31; 719:564–75.
27. Van Vollenhoven, R. F., Engleman, E. G., McGuire, J. L. An open study of dehydroepiandrosterone in systemic lupus erythematosus. *Arthritis Rheum* 1994 Sep; 37(9):1305–10.
28. Ambrosio, E., Casa, B., Bompasi, R., et al. Glucosamine sulphate: a controlled clinical investigation in arthrosis. *Pharmatherapeutica* 1981 2:504–8.
29. Pujalte, J. M., Llavore, E. P., Ylescupidez, F. R. Double-blind clinical evaluation of oral glucosamine sulphate in the basic treatment of osteoarthrosis. *Curr Med Res Opin* 1980 7:110–14.
30. Vaz, A. L. Double-blind clinical evaluation of the relative efficacy of ibuprofen and glucosamine sulphate in the management of osteoarthrosis of the knee in out-patients. *Curr Med Res Opin* 1982 8:145–49.
31. Uebelhart, D., Thonar, E. J., Delmas, P. D., Chantraine, A., Vignon, E. Effects of oral chondroitin sulfate on the progression of knee osteoarthritis: a pilot study. *Osteoarthritis Cartilage* 1998 May; 6 Suppl A:39–46.
32. Verbruggen, G., Goemaere, S., Veys, E. M. Chondroitin sulfate: S/DMOAD (structure/disease modifying anti-osteoarthritis drug) in the treatment of finger joint OA. *Osteoarthritis Cartilage* 1998 May; 6 Suppl A:37–38.
33. Bourgeois, P., Chales, G., Dehais, J., et al. Efficacy and tolerability of chondroitin sulfate 1200 mg/day vs chondroitin sulfate 3 x 400 mg/day vs placebo. *Osteoarthritis Cartilage* 1998 May; 6 Suppl A:25–30.
34. Kovacs, A. B. Efficacy of ipriflavone in the prevention and treatment of postmenopausal osteoporosis. *Agents Actions* 1994 Mar; 41(1–2):86–87.

35. Arjmandi, B. H., et al. The synthetic phytoestrogen, ipriflavone, and estrogen prevent bone loss by different mechanisms. *Calcif Tissue Int* 2000 Jan; 66(1):61–65.
36. Fujita, T., Fujii, Y., Miyauchi, A., Takagi, Y. Comparison of antiresorptive activities of ipriflavone, an isoflavone derivative, and elcatonin, an eel carbocalcitonin. *J Bone Miner Metab* 1999; 17(4):289–95.
37. Agnusdei, D., Bufalino, L. Efficacy of ipriflavone in established osteoporosis and long-term safety. *Calcif Tissue Int* 1997; 61 Suppl 1:S23–27.
38. Agnusdei, D., et al. Effects of ipriflavone on bone mass and calcium metabolism in postmenopausal osteoporosis. *Bone Miner* 1992 Oct; 19 Suppl 1:S43–48.
39. Passeri, M., et al. Effect of ipriflavone on bone mass in elderly osteoporotic women. *Bone Miner* 1992 Oct; 19 Suppl 1:S57–62.
40. Clements, M. L., Levine, M. M., Ristaino, P. A., Daya, V. E., Hughes, T. P. Exogenous lactobacilli fed to man—their fate and ability to prevent diarrheal disease. *Prog Food Nutr Sci* 1983; 7(3–4):29–37.
41. Shornikova, A. V., Casas, I. A., Mykkanen, H., Salo, E., Vesikari, T. Bacteriotherapy with Lactobacillus reuteri in rotavirus gastroenteritis. *Pediatr Infect Dis J* 1997 Dec; 16(12):1103–7.
42. Gorbach, S. L. Lactic acid bacteria and human health. *Ann Med* 1990 Feb; 22(1):37–41.
43. Rani, B., Khetarpaul, N. Probiotic fermented food mixtures: possible applications in clinical anti-diarrhoea usage. *Nutr Health* 1998; 12(2):97–105.
44. Ayebo, A. D., Shahani, K. M., Dam, R. Antitumor component(s) of yogurt: fractionation. *J Dairy Sci* 1981 Dec; 64(12):2318–23.
45. Yokokura, T., Kato, I., Matsuzaki, T., Mutai, M., Satoh, H. Antitumor activity of Lactobacillus casei YIT 9018 (LC 9018)—effect of administration route. *Gan To Kagaku Ryoho* 1984 Nov; 11(11):2427–33.
46. Goldin, B. R., Gorbach, S. L. Effect of Lactobacillus acidophilus dietary supplements on 1,2-dimethylhydrazine dihydrochloride-induced intestinal cancer in rats. *J Natl Cancer Inst* 1980 Feb; 64(2):263–65.

47. Lidbeck, A., Nord, C. E., Gustafsson, J. A., Rafter, J. Lactobacilli, anticarcinogenic activities and human intestinal microflora. *Eur J Cancer Prev* 1992 Aug; 1(5):341–53.

48. Rangavajhyala, N., Shahani, K. M., Sridevi, G., Srikumaran, S. Non-lipopolysaccharide component(s) of Lactobacillus acidophilus stimulate(s) the production of interleukin-1 alpha and tumor necrosis factor-alpha by murine macrophages. *Nutr Cancer* 1997; 28(2):130–34.

49. Ou, P., et al. Thioctic (lipoic acid): a therapeutic metal-chelating antioxidant? *Biochemical Pharmacology* 1995; 50(1):123–126.

50. Cameron, N. E., Cotter, M. A., Horrobin, D. H., Tritschler, H. J. Effects of alpha-lipoic acid on neurovascular function in diabetic rats: interaction with essential fatty acids. *Diabetologia* 1998 Apr; 41(4):390–99.

51. Ziegler, D., Gries, F. A. Alpha-lipoic acid in the treatment of diabetic peripheral and cardiac autonomic neuropathy. *Diabetes* 1997 Sep; 46 Suppl 2:S62–66.

52. Packer, L., Tritschler, H. J., Wessel, K. Neuroprotection by the metabolic antioxidant alpha-lipoic acid. *Free Radic Biol Med* 1997 22(1–2):359–78.

53. Skwarlo-Sonta, K. Functional connections between the pineal gland and immune system. *Acta Neurobiol Exp* (Warsz) 1996; 56(1):341–57.

54. Hakola, T., Harma, M. I., Laitinen, J. T. Circadian adjustment of men and women to night work. *Scand J Work Environ Health* 1996 Apr; 22(2):133–38.

55. Deacon, S., and Arendt, J. Adapting to phase shifts, I. An experimental model for jet lag and shift work. *Physiol Behav* 1996 Apr–May; 59(4–5):665–73.

56. Deacon, S., Arendt, J. Adapting to phase shifts, II. Effects of melatonin and conflicting light treatment. *Physiol Behav* 1996 Apr–May; 59(4–5):675–82.

57. Ronco, A. L., Halberg, F. The pineal gland and cancer. *Anticancer Res* 1996 Jul–Aug; 16(4A):2033–39.

58. Garcia-Patterson, A., Puig-Domingo, M., Webb, S. M. Thirty years of human pineal research: do we know its clinical relevance? *J Pineal Res* 1996 Jan; 20(1):1–6.

59. Conti, A., and Maestroni, G. J. The clinical neuroimmunotherapeutic role of melatonin in oncology. *J Pineal Res* 1995 Oct; 19(3):103–10.
60. Acuna-Castroviejo, D., Escames, G., et al. Cell protective role of melatonin in the brain. *J Pineal Res* 1995 Sep; 19(2):57–63.
61. Reiter, R. J. The role of the neurohormone melatonin as a buffer against macromolecular oxidative damage. *Neurochem Int* 1995 Dec; 27(6):453–60.
62. Daniels, W. M., Reiter, R. J., Melchiorri, D., et al. Melatonin counteracts lipid peroxidation induced by carbon tetrachloride but does not restore glucose-6 phosphatase activity. *J Pineal Res* 1995 Aug; 19(1):1–6.
63. Viviani, S., Negretti, E., Orazi, A., et al. Preliminary studies on melatonin in the treatment of myelodysplastic syndromes following cancer chemotherapy. *J Pineal Res* 1990; 8(4):347–54.
64. Jacob, S. W., Herschler, R. Dimethyl sulfoxide after twenty years. *Ann N Y Acad Sci* 1983; 411:xiii–xvii.
65. Brown, J. H., Wood, D. C., Jacob, S. W. Current status of dimethyl sulfoxide (DMSO). A double blind evaluation of its therapeutic value in acute strains, sprains, bursitis and tendonitis. *Bull Soc Int Chir* 1972 Nov–Dec; 31(6):561–66.
66. Murav'ev, IuV., et al. [Effect of dimethyl sulfoxide and dimethyl sulfone on a destructive process in the joints of mice with spontaneous arthritis]. *Patol Fiziol Eksp Ter* 1991 Mar–Apr; (2):37–39.
67. Beilke, M. A., Collins-Lech, C., Sohnle, P. G. Effects of dimethyl sulfoxide on the oxidative function of human neutrophils. *J Lab Clin Med* 1987 Jul; 110(1):91–96.
68. Layman, D. L. Growth inhibitory effects of dimethyl sulfoxide and dimethyl sulfone on vascular smooth muscle and endothelial cells in vitro. *In Vitro Cell Dev Biol* 1987 Jun; 23(6):422–28.
69. Farina, C., Fiori, M. G., Crepaldi, G. Cognitive decline in the elderly: a double-blind, placebo-controlled multicenter study on efficacy of phosphatidylserine administration. *Aging* 1993; 5:123–33.
70. Crook, T., Petrie, W., Wells, C., Massari, D. C. Effects of phosphatidylserine in Alzheimer's disease. *Psychopharmacol Bull* 1992; 28:61–66.

71. Crook, T. H., Tinklenberg, J., Yesavage, J., et al. Effects of phosphatidylserine in age-associated memory impairment. *Neurology* 1991; 41:644–49.
72. Maggioni, M., Picotti, G. B., Bondiolotti, G. P., et al. Effects of phosphatidylserine therapy in geriatric patients with depressive disorders. *Acta Psychiatr Scand* 1990; 81:265–70.
73. Delwaide, P. J., Gyselynck-Mambourg, A. M., Hurlet, A., Ylieff, M. Double-blind randomized controlled study of phosphatidylserine in senile demented patients. *Acta Neurol Scand* 1986; 73:136–40.
74. Navarro Cruz, D., et al. [Transference factor in moderate and severe atopic dermatitis]. *Rev Alerg Mex* 1996 Sep–Oct; 43(5):116–23.
75. Estrada-Parra, S., et al. Comparative study of transfer factor and acyclovir in the treatment of herpes zoster. *Int J Immunopharmacol* 1998 Oct; 20(10):521–35.
76. Hana, I., Vrubel, J., Pekarek, J., Cech, K. The influence of age on transfer factor treatment of cellular immunodeficiency, chronic fatigue syndrome and/or chronic viral infections. *Biotherapy* 1996; 9(1–3):91–95.
77. Whyte, R. I., Schork, M. A., Sloan, H., Orringer, M. B., Kirsh, M. M. Adjuvant treatment using transfer factor for bronchogenic carcinoma: long-term follow-up. *Ann Thorac Surg* 1992 Mar; 53(3):391–96.
78. Ferrer-Argote, V. E., et al. Successful treatment of severe complicated measles with non-specific transfer factor. *In Vivo* 1994 Jul–Aug; 8(4):555–57.
79. Pizza, G., De Vinci, C., Cuzzocrea, D., et al. A preliminary report on the use of transfer factor for treating stage D3 hormone-unresponsive metastatic prostate cancer. *Biotherapy* 1996; 9(1–3):123–32.
80. De Vinci, C., Pizza, G., Cuzzocrea, D., et al. Use of transfer factor for the treatment of recurrent non-bacterial female cystitis (NBRC): a preliminary report. *Biotherapy* 1996; 9(1–3):133–38.

Chapter 10. Practical Guidelines: Buying and Taking Supplements

1. Businco, L., Falconieri, P., Giampietro, P., Bellioni, B. Food allergy and asthma. *Pediatr Pulmonol Suppl* 1995; 11:59–60.
2. Sicherer, S. H. Manifestations of food allergy: evaluation and management. *Am Fam Physician* 1999 Jan 15; 59(2):415–24, 429–30.

3. Beri, D., Malaviya, A. N., Shandilya, R., Singh, R. R. Effect of dietary restrictions on disease activity in rheumatoid arthritis. *Ann Rheum Dis* 1988 Jan; 47(1):69–72.
4. Kjeldsen-Kragh, J., and Haugen, M., et al. Controlled trial of fasting and one-year vegetarian diet in rheumatoid arthritis. *Lancet* 1991 Oct 12; 338(8772):899–902.
5. Adam, O. Nutrition as adjuvant therapy in chronic polyarthritis. *Z Rheumatol* 1993 Sep–Oct; 52(5):275–80.
6. Mathew, N. T. Kurman, R., Perez, F. Drug induced refractory headache—clinical features and management. *Headache* 1990 Oct; 30(10):634–38.
7. Mathew, N. T. Chronic refractory headache. *Neurology* 1993 Jun; 43(6 Suppl 3):S26–33.
8. Walker, J., Parisi, S., Olive, D. Analgesic rebound headache: experience in a community hospital. *South Med J* 1993 Nov; 86(11):1202–5.
9. Rapoport, A., Stang, P., et al. Analgesic rebound headache in clinical practice: data from a physician survey. *Headache* 1996 Jan; 36(1):14–19.
10. Symon, D. N. Twelve cases of analgesic headache. *Arch Dis Child* 1998 Jun; 78(6):555–56.

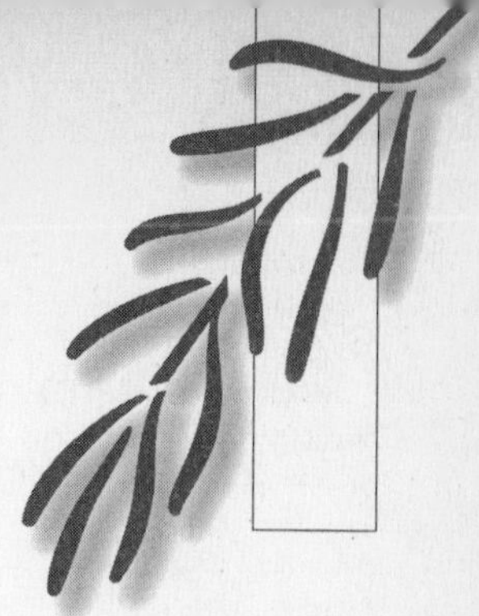

Index

MICHAEL JANSON, M.D., received his medical degree from Boston University in 1970. He practices preventive and alternative medicine in the Boston area, and has been recommending dietary supplements in his clinical practice since 1976. A past president of both the American Preventive Medical Association and the American College for Advancement in Medicine, and a charter member of the American Holistic Medical Association, Dr. Janson is a member of the National Speakers Association, and he speaks internationally on the subjects of healthy lifestyles, nutrition, alternative medicine, and dietary supplements. He has twice testified before U.S. Senate committees on dietary supplements and alternative medicine. In addition to his lecturing, Dr. Janson teaches in the anti-aging workshops of the American College for Advancement in Medicine, and regularly writes articles for magazines and professional journals. He is a frequent radio and television guest, and has hosted his own radio health show.